the no excuses cookbook

Michelle Bridges became a household name when she first appeared as a trainer on Channel Ten's hit reality weight-loss show *The Biggest Loser*. She is now Australia's most recognised personal trainer, having working in the fitness and weight-loss industry for over two decades. Michelle is a nationally recognised spokesperson for brands and causes close to her heart and is hugely sought after as a motivational speaker.

The No Excuses Cookbook is her fifth book. *Crunch TIme, Crunch Time Cookbook, Losing the Last 5 Kilos* and *5 Minutes a Day* were bestsellers. *Losing the Last 5 Kilos* debuted at number 1 nationally.

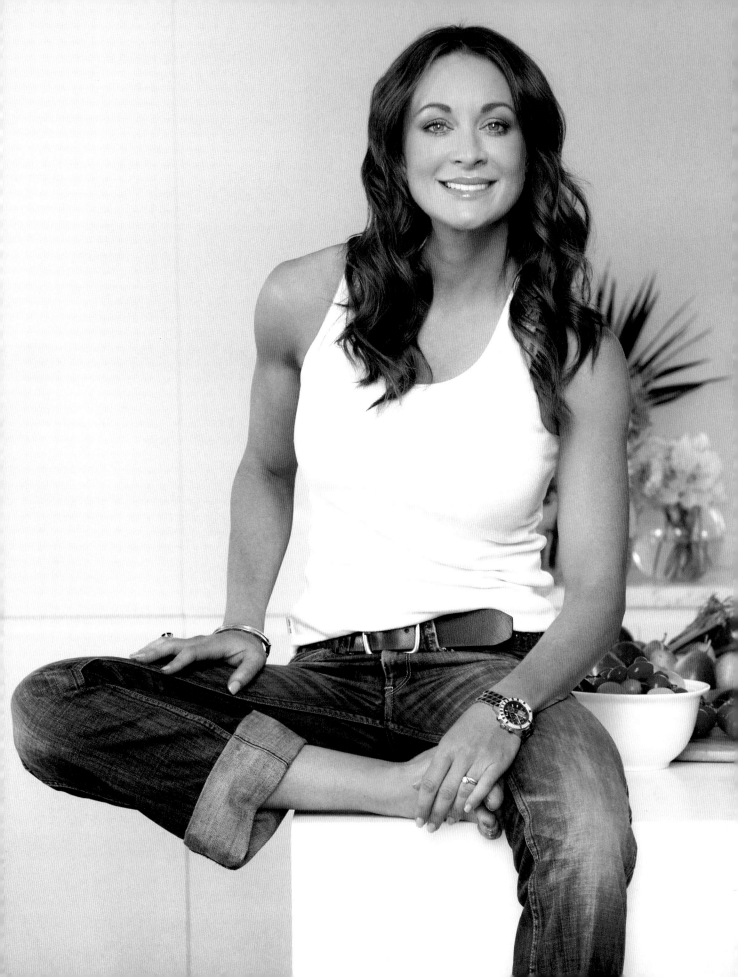

the no excuses cookbook

weight-loss recipes
for *everyday life*

michelle bridges

VIKING
an imprint of
PENGUIN BOOKS

For my mum

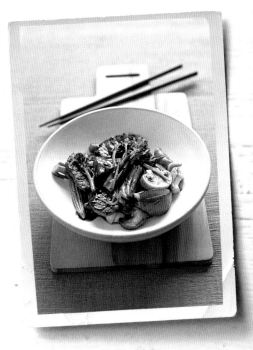

VIKING

Published by the Penguin Group
Penguin Group (Australia)
250 Camberwell Road, Camberwell, Victoria 3124, Australia
(a division of Pearson Australia Group Pty Ltd)
Penguin Group (USA) Inc.
375 Hudson Street, New York, New York 10014, USA
Penguin Group (Canada)
90 Eglinton Avenue East, Suite 700, Toronto, Canada ON M4P 2Y3
(a division of Pearson Penguin Canada Inc.)
Penguin Books Ltd
80 Strand, London WC2R 0RL, England
Penguin Ireland
25 St Stephen's Green, Dublin 2, Ireland
(a division of Penguin Books Ltd)
Penguin Books India Pvt Ltd
11 Community Centre, Panchsheel Park, New Delhi – 110 017, India
Penguin Group (NZ)
67 Apollo Drive, Rosedale, North Shore 0632, New Zealand
(a division of Pearson New Zealand Ltd)
Penguin Books (South Africa) (Pty) Ltd
24 Sturdee Avenue, Rosebank, Johannesburg 2196, South Africa

Penguin Books Ltd, Registered Offices: 80 Strand, London WC2R 0RL, England

First published by Penguin Group (Australia), 2012

10 9 8 7 6 5 4 3 2 1

Cover and text design by Adam Laszczuk © Penguin Group (Australia)
Cover and author photographs by Nick Wilson
Food photography by Julie Renouf, home economy by Caroline Jones, food styling by Georgia Young
The publisher would like to thank Exlibris Prints, Market Import and Safari Living for providing materials for the food photography.
Typeset in Fonce Sans Pro by Post Pre-Press Group, Brisbane, Queensland
Colour reproduction by Splitting Image, Clayton, Victoria
Printed and bound in China by South China Printing Co Ltd

National Library of Australia
Cataloguing-in-Publication data:

Bridges, Michelle.

The no excuses cookbook : weight-loss recipes for everyday life / Michelle Bridges.
9780670076376 (pbk.)
Includes index.
Reducing diets--Recipes. Reducing diets. Nutrition--Requirements.

641.5635

penguin.com.au

While every care has been taken in researching and compiling the dietary and exercise information in this book,
it is in no way intended to replace or supersede professional medical advice. Neither the author nor the publisher
may be held responsible for any action or claim howsoever resulting from the use of this book or any information
contained in it. Readers must obtain their own professional medical advice before relying on or otherwise making
use of the dietary and exercise information in this book

Contents

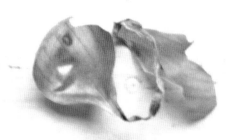

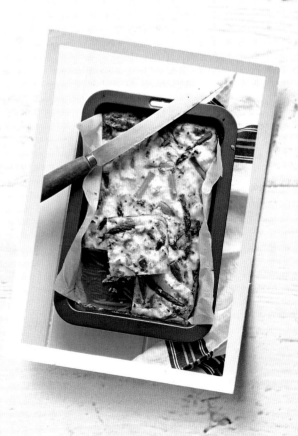

Introduction

What you eat is even more important than how much exercise you do. I've said it before, but it's worth saying again: your weight and your health will always come down to what you put in your mouth. So it's super-essential to eat well – not just while you're torching the extra kilos, but for the rest of your life. (Of course, exercise is still important – good for the body and equally good for the head!)

If you've read any of my other books, though, you'll know I'm not about deprivation or eating food that tastes like cardboard. Eating for good health should be fun! And learning to cook good, nutritious food for yourself is not only a big money-saver, it's one of the most important skills you can have for your health and one of the best gifts you could pass on to your kids. Plus, you can put together a great meal in the time it would take you to get takeaway – promise! It's time to stop eating like a teenager and start taking control of what goes into your body. No excuses.

That's where this book comes in: it's packed with simple, nutritious recipes that taste brilliant and will keep you on the straight and narrow weight-wise. Just remember a few basic food rules:

Watch your calories. Remember, eat more than you burn and you'll put on weight. The dishes in this book clock in at between 250 and 350 calories per serve, so three meals a day plus snacks will hit most people's recommended daily intake, no problems. To lose weight, women need to stick to 1200 calories a day, and men to 1800 calories – check out the menu plan at the back of the book for some example days.

Keep an eye on the scales. If the kilos are starting to creep up and you're having to jump around the room to zip up your favourite jeans, take action. Check your portion sizes and calorie counts, cut back on the alcohol and ramp up your exercise.

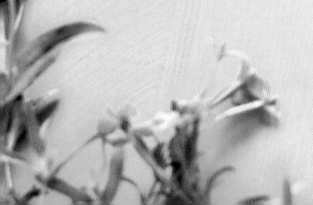

Set limits for yourself. Use smaller plates, *never* go back for seconds, *never* eat while you're cooking, and *never* eat the leftovers.

Dessert is a luxury. You'll see I've put in a few dessert recipes, but I don't want you to get the wrong idea and eat them every day – they're for special occasions *only*, people! Don't let your sweet tooth destroy all your hard work.

Eat whole foods – the fresher the better!

Consider how what you eat affects others. I take a strong stance on only eating ethically produced, organic and free-range meat, fish and produce: better for you, better for the environment, and definitely better for the animals you eat. Take a look at 'Food values' on page 26 for more.

Make eating well automatic. If you learn a handful of great recipes, put together a quick plan each week and shop to your plan, then you'll never be tempted to pick up pizza on the way home or eat a whole packet of biscuits as 'dinner'. If you've never cooked before, choose just two or three of the simplest recipes to start with, to get your confidence up. You'll be branching out in no time.

The beauty of this book is that it has recipes for all events – from picnics to parties, and breakfast to barbecues. To be straight with you, this isn't a diet book, it's a book for everyday meals that I'm sure you'll love as much as I do.

The great flavours mean that the recipes are super-tasty, totally yum and satisfying.

Happy cooking!

Michelle xoxo

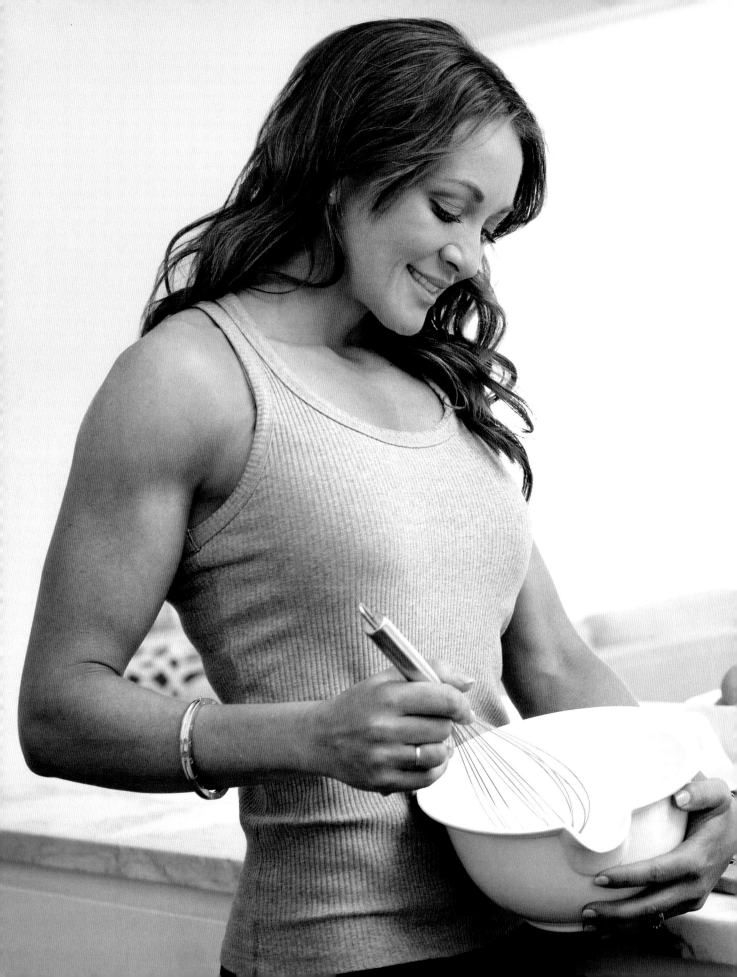

breakfast

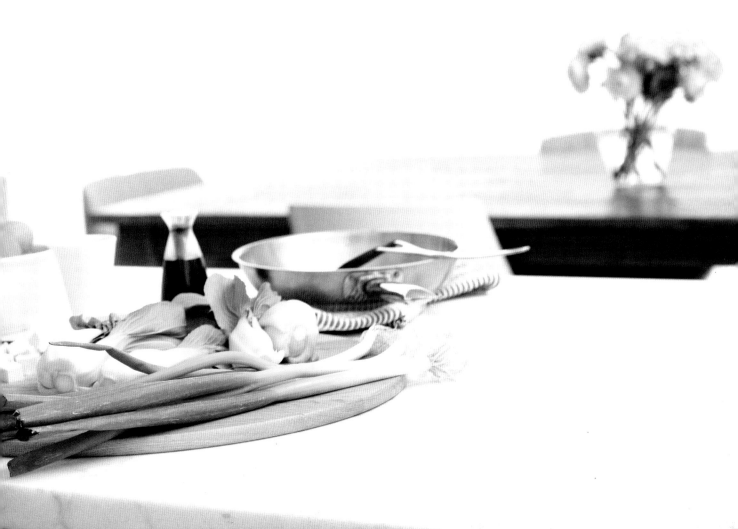

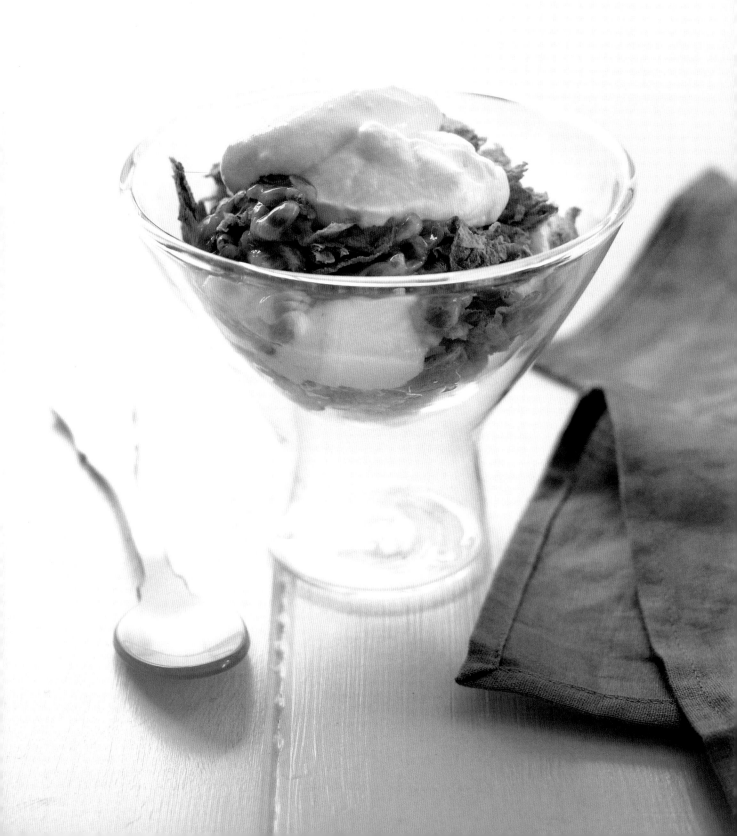

Morning Weet-Bix and passionfruit trifle

Trifle for breakfast? Sure! Thick, plain yoghurt plus tangy passionfruit make this brekkie really luscious as well as nutritious.

SERVES 2 | **PREP** 2 minutes | **CAL PER SERVE** 342

6 fresh passionfruit
8 Weet-Bix biscuits
1 cup plain low-cal yoghurt

1. Remove the pulp from the passionfruit and discard the skins.

2. Break four of the biscuits roughly (just enough to form a layer) and divide between two glass bowls. Top with half of the yoghurt and passionfruit.

3. Repeat the layers with the remaining ingredients and serve immediately so the biscuits are still crunchy.

TIP: This breakfast is also great with half sliced strawberries and half passionfruit.

Sweet couscous with orange juice and dried fruit

For the sweet tooths out there. A warm, filling breakfast really sets you up for the day: this couscous can be made in a snap and gives you your daily serves of fruit as well. Give it a try!

SERVES 2 | PREP 10 minutes | COOK 2 minutes | CAL PER SERVE 353

½ cup freshly squeezed orange juice
⅓ cup couscous
60 g dried figs, diced
40 g pitted prunes, diced

¼ cup currants
½ cup plain low-cal yoghurt
pinch of ground cinnamon

1. Heat the orange juice in a small saucepan until hot (do not boil). Pour the hot juice over the couscous in a medium bowl and stir well. Stand, covered, for 2 minutes, then stir again. Repeat until fluffy. Stir the dried fruit through.

2. Serve the couscous with a dollop of yoghurt and a sprinkle of cinnamon.

TIP: You can store any leftover couscous and fruit in an airtight container in the fridge. Just warm it up in the microwave on medium before adding the yoghurt and cinnamon.

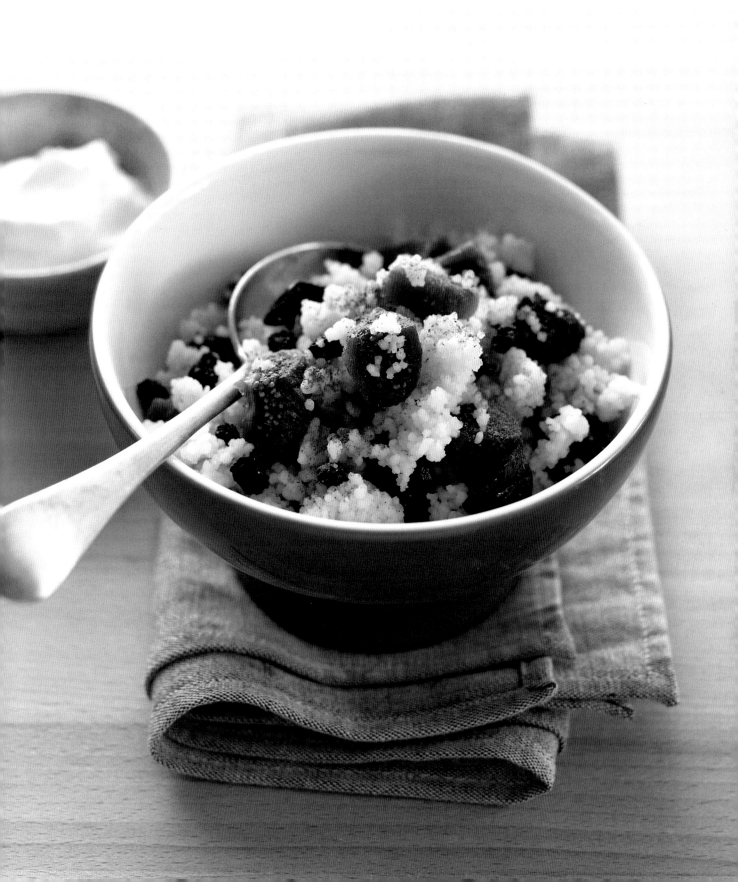

All-Bran fruit salad

This cereal-and-fruit combo is an absolute basic that you could eat every day – and it'll make breakfast a treat every time.

SERVES 2 | **PREP** 10 minutes | **CAL PER SERVE** 350

1⅓ cups All-Bran or similar cereal
200 g rockmelon, peeled, seeded
   and cut into chunks
200 g honeydew melon, peeled,
   seeded and cut into chunks

200 g seedless grapes, halved if large
1 small banana, peeled and sliced
½ cup low-cal milk

1. Divide the bran between two bowls, then top it with equal serves of the fruit and ¼ cup of milk each.

TIP: Toasted muesli is a delicious alternative to the All-Bran in this recipe, but it's more calorie-dense, so you only need to use ½ cup in each bowl.

Apple and pear porridge with cinnamon

The apple and pear add a delicious twist to this porridge.
Great after a morning workout in winter!

SERVES 2 | PREP 10 minutes | COOK 10 minutes | CAL PER SERVE 332

1 cup rolled oats
2 tablespoons sultanas
1 large pear, cored

1 large green apple, coarsely grated
pinch of ground cinnamon

1. Place the oats, sultanas and 2 cups of water into a small saucepan and bring it to the boil, then reduce the heat to low and cook the porridge for 5 minutes, stirring occasionally.

2. Meanwhile, dice half of the pear and slice the rest.

3. Stir the grated apple and diced pear into the porridge. Divide between two bowls, top with the sliced pear and sprinkle with cinnamon.

TIP: You don't need to peel the apple or pear in this recipe – the skins add some extra crunch and fibre.

White beans with spinach on toast

This is the perfect dish for a weekend brunch with friends; it also makes a great, quick Sunday-night meal when you don't feel like cooking.

SERVES 4 | **PREP** 10 minutes | **COOK** 10 minutes | **CAL PER SERVE** 342

olive oil spray
4 eggs
2 teaspoons olive oil
1 brown onion, diced
1 clove garlic, crushed
2 × 420 g cans cannellini beans,
   drained and rinsed

8 slices mixed-grain bread
80 g baby spinach
1 large tomato, diced
⅓ cup shaved parmesan

1. Lightly spray a large non-stick frying pan with olive oil and heat on medium–high. Break the eggs into the pan and cook for 1–2 minutes until the whites are set, then slide them out onto 4 warm plates.

2. Heat the olive oil in a large saucepan on medium and cook the onion and garlic, stirring, for 5 minutes or until softened. Stir in the beans and cook until heated through; meanwhile, put the bread in the toaster. Add the spinach and tomato to the bean mixture, stir, and cook until the spinach is just wilted.

3. Add two pieces of toast to the egg on each plate, and spoon over the beans. Top with the parmesan and serve immediately.

TIP: If you're only serving two people, try making the full quantity anyway and using the leftover bean mixture to make a dip for your lunch box. Simply place it in a food processor with ¼ cup plain low-cal yoghurt and a tablespoon each of tahini and lemon juice and process until smooth. It's delicious served with carrot, cucumber and celery sticks and a small wholemeal pita bread, toasted. (If you chop 100 g of each of the vegetable sticks, it's 251 cal per serve for two people.)

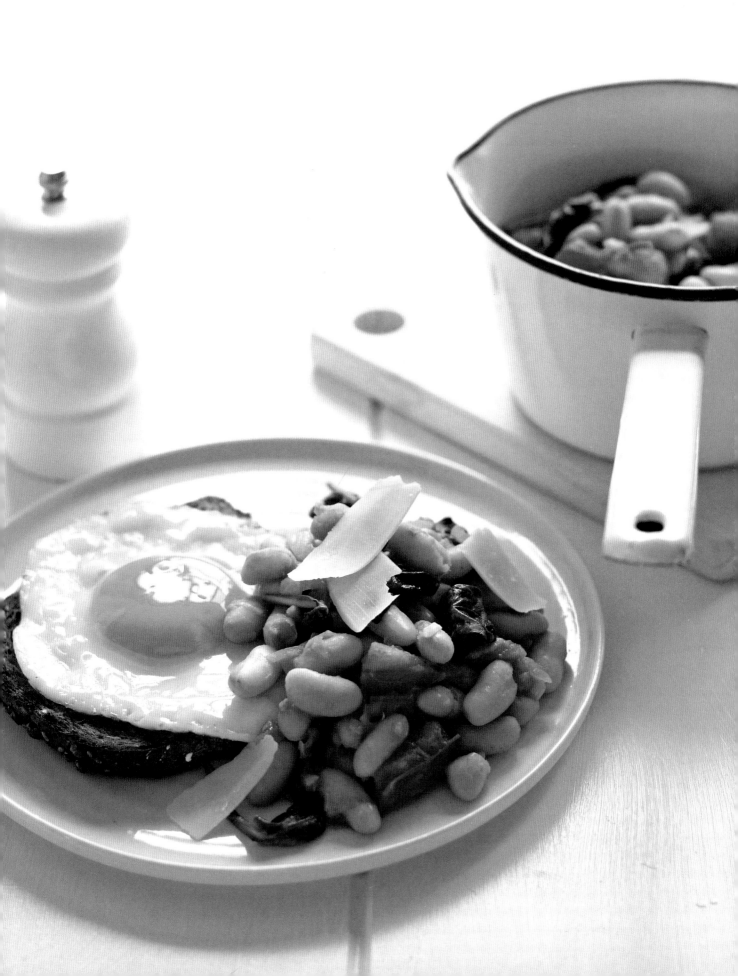

Turkey and egg toastie

Skip the cafe stop and take this toastie to eat at work instead. The turkey makes a delicious change from the usual ham and cheese.

SERVES 2 | PREP 5 minutes | COOK 10 minutes | CAL PER SERVE 335

olive oil spray
4 slices wholemeal bread
2 eggs
80 g shaved turkey

⅓ cup grated low-cal cheddar
1 small tomato, sliced
2 teaspoons Dijon mustard

1. Preheat a flat sandwich press and lightly spray it with olive oil.

2. Cut a 4 cm circle out of the centre of two of the slices of bread and discard the circles. Place the slices in the sandwich press, break an egg into each hole and cook for 2–3 minutes until the egg white starts to set. Top with turkey, cheddar and tomato. Spread the remaining slices of bread with mustard and place them on top, mustard-side down, then bring down the sandwich-maker's lid to toast the tops. Be careful not to push them down too much, or the eggs will break and spill out. Cook for another 2–3 minutes and serve immediately.

TIP: If you don't have a sandwich press, you can use a non-stick frying pan. Wait until the egg is set, then add the filling and the top slice of bread and flip the sandwich to toast it on the other side, pressing down gently with a spatula.

Omelette stir-fry with tofu and bok choy

I love omelettes for a quick and tasty hit of protein in the morning.
Fantastic for a leisurely brunch with the weekend papers, too!

SERVES 2 | PREP 10 minutes | COOK 5 minutes | CAL PER SERVE 357

1 teaspoon peanut oil
6 spring onions, coarsely chopped
   on the diagonal
1 clove garlic, thinly sliced
5 eggs, lightly beaten

¼ cup good-quality chicken stock
1 teaspoon low-salt soy sauce
1 bunch baby bok choy, leaves
   separated and coarsely chopped
150 g firm tofu, cut into 1 cm cubes

1. Heat the peanut oil in a non-stick wok on high and stir-fry the spring onion and garlic for 2 minutes until charred and softened. Remove them from the wok.

2. Pour the eggs into the wok, swirling them to make an omelette. Cook for 1 minute until starting to set, then stir-fry the omelette to break it into large chunks. Return the spring onion and garlic to the wok, add the stock, soy sauce, bok choy and tofu, and stir-fry until the leaves start to wilt. Serve immediately.

TIP: If you're not a fan of tofu, feel free to leave it out and serve the stir-fry with 2 slices of toasted wholemeal bread – a 'fusion breakfast'! (328 cal per serve.)

Corn fritters

Corn fritters are a staple of the cafe brekkie, but they're super-easy to make at home. The fresh corn kernels just burst with sweetness in your mouth.

SERVES 2 | PREP 10 minutes | COOK 20 minutes | CAL PER SERVE 357

1 fresh corncob
2 medium eggs
½ cup wholemeal self-raising flour
½ cup low-cal milk

1 spring onion, finely chopped
olive oil spray
2 tablespoons mint leaves

1. Place the corncob upright on a board and cut away the kernels.

2. Whisk the eggs in a large bowl with a fork. Stir in the corn kernels, flour, milk and half of the spring onion.

3. Lightly spray a large non-stick frying pan with olive oil and heat on medium–high. Drop heaped ¼ cup measures of the egg mixture into the pan, in batches, to make 6 fritters, and flatten each with the back of a spoon. Fry for 3–4 minutes on each side until golden and cooked through.

4. Serve immediately, sprinkled with the mint leaves and remaining spring onion.

TIPS: Make sure you flatten the fritters well, as if they're too thick they won't cook through properly.

• You can also use canned corn for this dish: you'll need 2 × 125 g cans corn kernels, drained and rinsed.

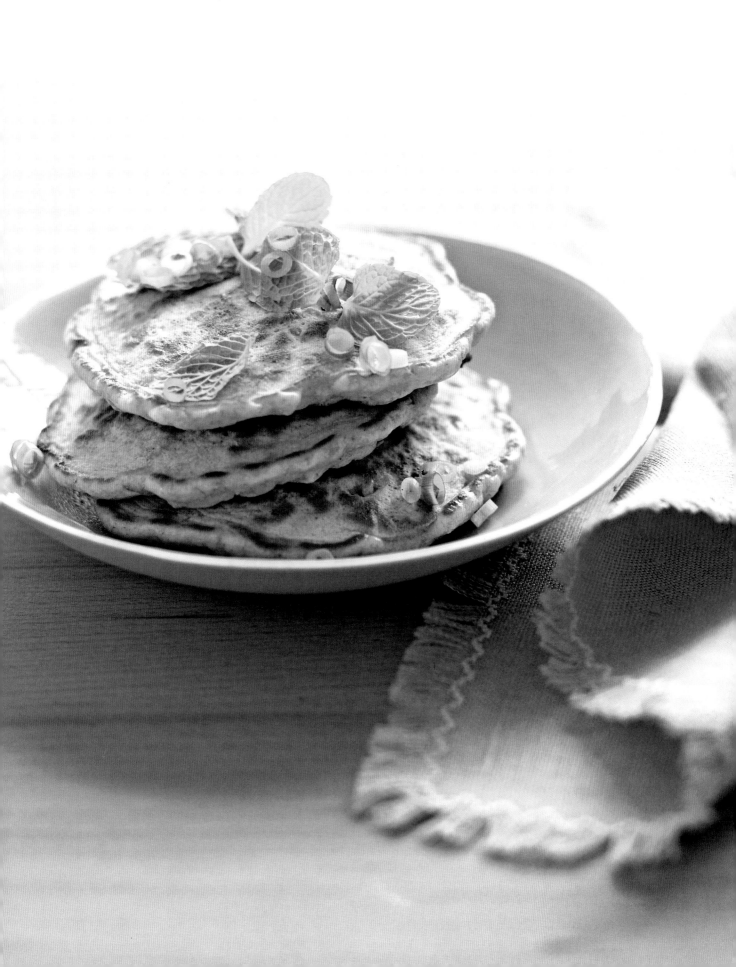

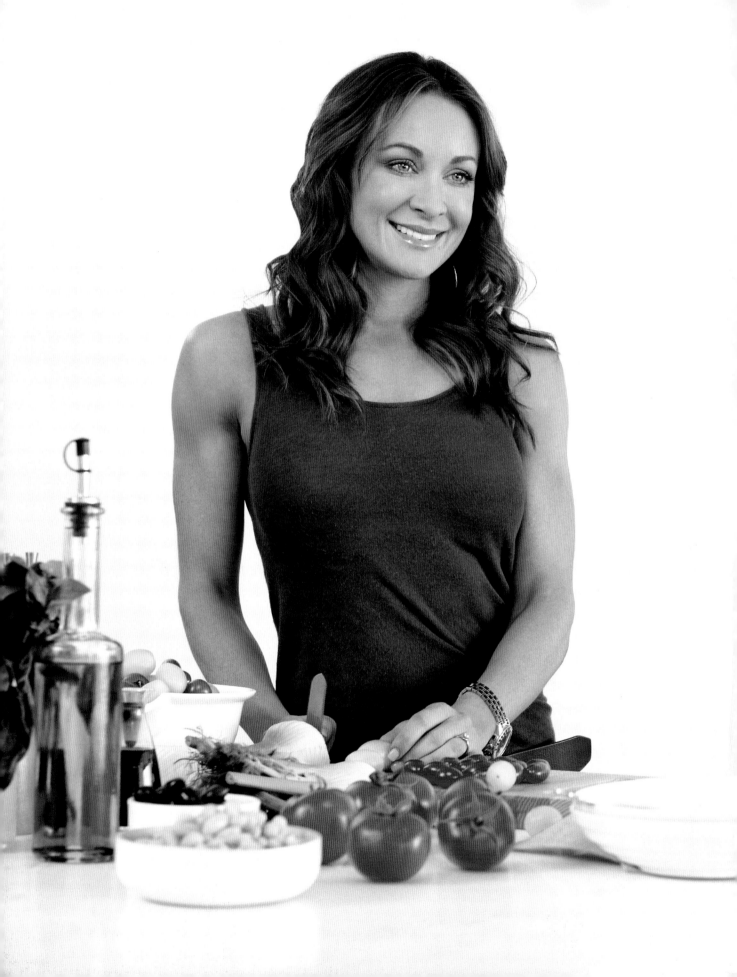

lunch

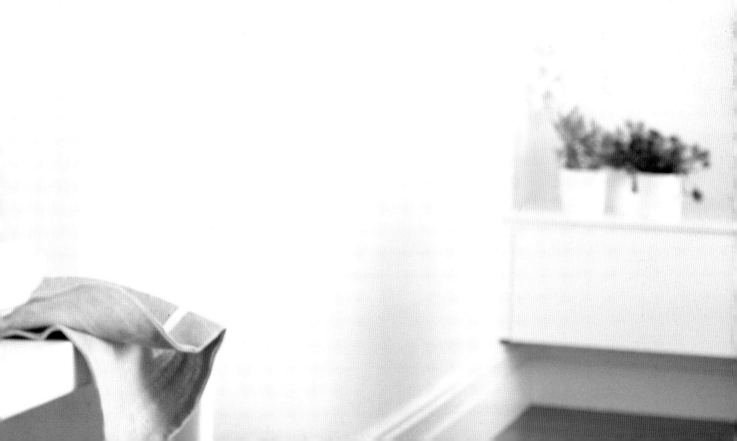

Egg and tarragon sandwich

Tarragon and chilli make this egg sandwich something special.
A traditional accompaniment to eggs in French cooking, fresh
tarragon is available in most supermarkets during summer.
(If you can't find it, chervil is a good substitute.)

SERVES 2 | PREP 10 minutes | COOK 10 minutes | CAL PER SERVE 320

3 large eggs
¼ cup low-cal ricotta
¼ cup low-cal cottage cheese
1 spring onion, finely chopped

2 teaspoons finely chopped
   fresh tarragon
pinch of finely chopped red chilli
   (optional)
4 slices mixed-grain bread

1. Boil the eggs in a small saucepan for
   6 minutes, then place into cold water
   and peel when cool enough to handle.
   Once peeled, coarsely mash with the
   back of a fork in a medium bowl and
   stir in the ricotta, cottage cheese, spring
   onion, tarragon and chilli (if using) until
   combined.

2. Spread the mixture over 2 slices of the
   bread and top with the remaining slices.

TIP: You don't need much chilli to add
a zing to the sandwich – but if you love it,
go ahead and add more!

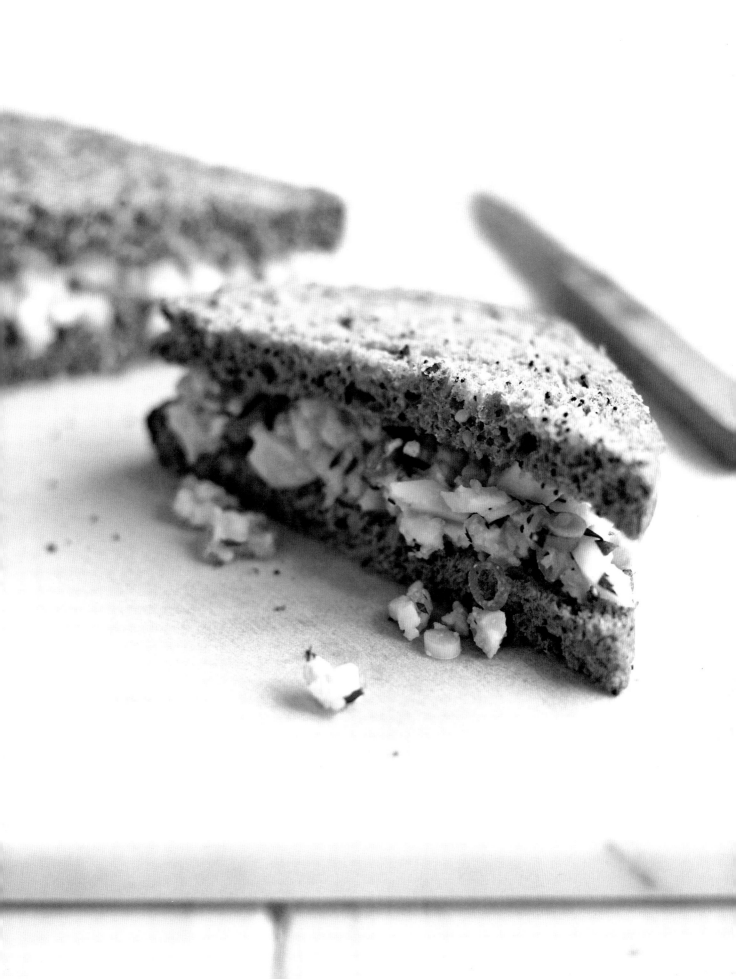

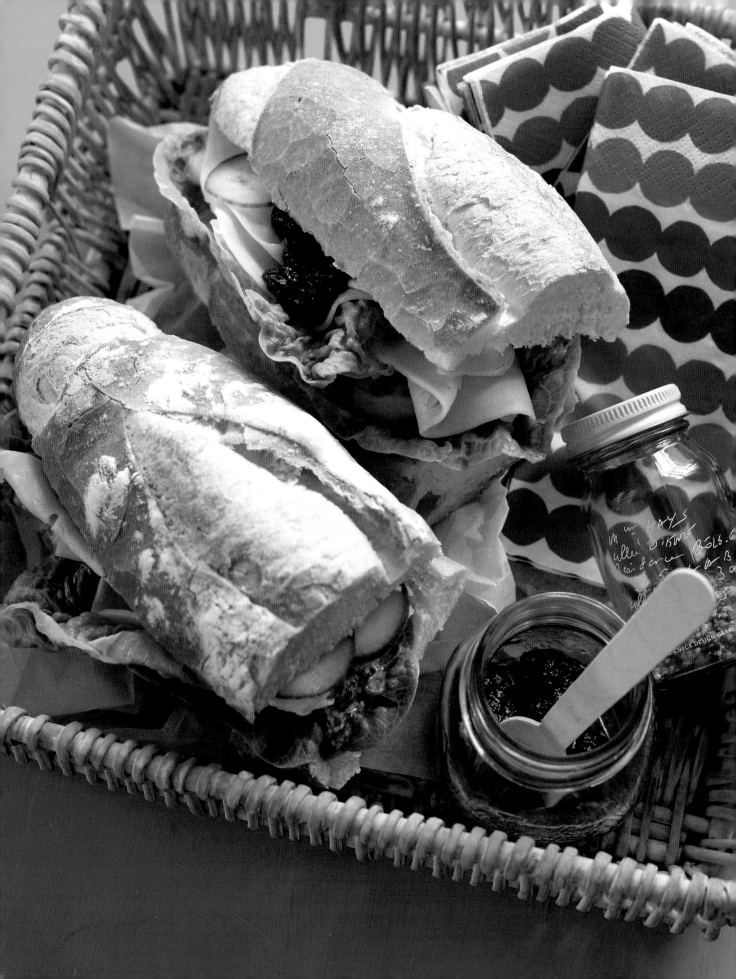

Turkey and cranberry sandwich

Sandwiches are a lunch staple, but they don't have to be boring. Turkey and cranberry in good bread is a satisfying combination.

SERVES 2 | PREP 5 minutes | CAL PER SERVE 323

½ small breadstick, halved widthwise
1½ tablespoons cranberry sauce
1 tablespoon wholegrain mustard

4 baby cos lettuce leaves
½ Lebanese cucumber, thinly sliced
80 g thinly sliced cooked turkey

1. Using a serrated knife, split the breadstick pieces open. Spread the bases with cranberry sauce and the tops with mustard, then fill with the lettuce, cucumber and turkey.

Lamb and tabouli pockets

Who needs a kebab shop when you can make these gorgeous pockets at home? If you're packing them for lunch, keep the pita bread separate and fill it when you're ready to eat so that it doesn't go soggy.

SERVES 2 | PREP 15 minutes | COOK 10 minutes | CAL PER SERVE 299

olive oil spray
120 g lamb backstrap
freshly ground black pepper
2 wholemeal pita pockets
   (11–15 cm wide)

Tabouli
¼ cup bulgur (cracked wheat)
1 ripe tomato, diced
½ Lebanese cucumber, diced
¼ red onion, diced
¼ cup finely chopped parsley
¼ cup finely chopped mint
2 teaspoons extra virgin olive oil
2 teaspoons lemon juice
freshly ground black pepper

1. To make the tabouli, cover the bulgur with boiling water and let stand for 10 minutes. Drain, rinse with cold water and drain again, then tip the bulgur into a clean tea towel and wring it out to dry. Place in a bowl with the remaining tabouli ingredients, season with pepper and toss to combine.

2. Meanwhile, lightly spray a medium frying pan or char-grill with olive oil and heat on high. Season the lamb with pepper, then cook for 2–3 minutes a side until well browned (or charred) but still pink inside. Stand for 2 minutes before slicing thinly.

3. Fill the pita pockets with the tabouli and sliced lamb.

TIPS: If you heat the pita pockets in the microwave to soften them, they will be less likely to tear when you open them.

• You could also double the tabouli and serve the leftovers as a side dish for 2 × 150 g grilled chicken breasts sprinkled with za'atar (serves 2 – 294 cal per serve).

Cucumber, feta and za'atar roll

A terrific wrap to take for lunch or a picnic. The za'atar spice mix adds an absolutely knockout aroma – you'll find yourself wanting to add it to everything!

SERVES 2 | PREP 10 minutes | CAL PER SERVE 277

4 pieces Mountain Bread
2 teaspoons za'atar
1 Lebanese cucumber, sliced
120 g low-cal feta, crumbled

1 spring onion, thinly sliced
100 g iceberg lettuce, shredded
¼ cup shredded mint

1. Place the pieces of bread on a clean board and sprinkle with za'atar. Divide the cucumber, feta, spring onion, lettuce and mint between the pieces, placing it at one end. Roll each piece tightly around the filling.

TIP: Za'atar is a Middle Eastern spice mix – its ingredients vary, but usually include sesame seeds, dried herbs (often thyme) and salt, and sometimes spices such as cumin and sumac. It's great to use as a rub for barbecued meat, or to add a zing to some toast with a bowl of soup.

Celeriac coleslaw and rare roast beef sandwich

Roast beef and celeriac is a fantastic flavour combination! It might not be pretty on the outside, but celeriac's distinctive taste works beautifully with the yoghurt, mustard and beef in this dish.

SERVES 2 | **PREP** 10 minutes | **CAL PER SERVE** 303

4 slices dark rye bread
80 g rare roast beef, sliced

Celeriac coleslaw
150 g celeriac, peeled
¼ cup plain low-cal yoghurt
1 tablespoon lemon juice
2 teaspoons Dijon mustard
freshly ground black pepper

1. To make the coleslaw, finely shred the celeriac and combine immediately with the yoghurt, lemon juice and mustard in a medium bowl. Season with pepper.

2. Spread 2 slices of the bread with half of the coleslaw, then top with the roast beef and the remaining coleslaw and bread.

TIP: For dinner, you could double the coleslaw quantities and serve it with 2 × 180 g grilled rump steaks (serves 2 – 303 cal per serve) or 2 × 150 g grilled salmon fillets, skin off (serves 2 – 284 cal per serve).

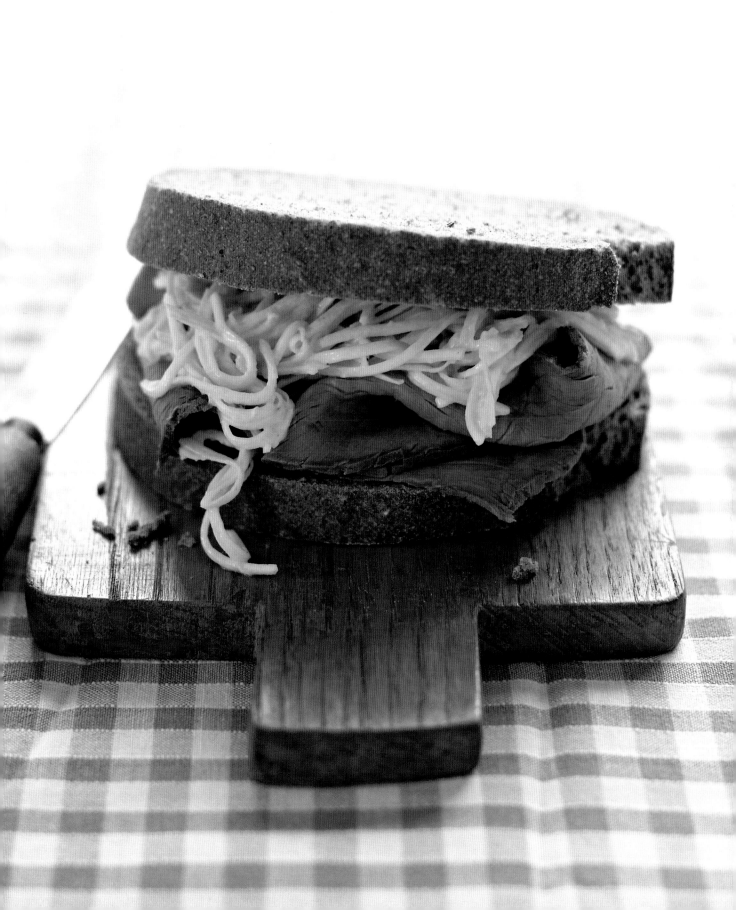

Chicken, beetroot and mint sandwich

Having a little cooked chicken in the fridge for a quick sandwich
is very handy. You can pan-fry several breast fillets on the weekend
(or poach them for moist, extra-tender meat, which is what I love to do).
Then you just need to shred or slice them on the day.

SERVES 2 | **PREP** 10 minutes | **CAL PER SERVE** 299

4 slices wholegrain bread
2 tablespoons wholegrain mustard
150 g cooked chicken breast, sliced

225 g can sliced beetroot, drained
⅓ cup torn mint leaves
freshly ground black pepper

1. Spread the bread with mustard. Top 2 slices
   with the chicken, beetroot and mint, and
   season with freshly ground black pepper.
   Cover with the remaining slices of bread,
   mustard-side down, and cut as desired.

Smoked salmon and strawberry salad

Smoked salmon is an everyday luxury that packs a great protein and omega-3 punch. This pretty salad will make your co-workers envious at lunch and add glamour to a picnic.

SERVES 2 | PREP 10 minutes | CAL PER SERVE 313

200 g smoked salmon, torn
250 g strawberries, hulled and halved
100 g mesclun salad mix
15 cm (40 g) breadstick, very thinly
  sliced on the diagonal and toasted

1 tablespoon extra virgin olive oil
2 teaspoons white balsamic vinegar
freshly ground black pepper

1. Combine the smoked salmon, strawberries, mesclun and toasted breadstick slices in a large bowl. Drizzle with the olive oil and vinegar, season, and toss to coat.

TIP: If you're packing this for a lunch box, keep the toasted breadstick and the dressing separate and assemble the salad when you're ready to eat, to keep everything crisp.

Food values

Since I wrote my first recipe book, *Crunch Time Cookbook*, there's been an avalanche of interest in restaurants, cooking and produce. Ten years ago it would have been hard to imagine, but our fascination with food isn't showing signs of going away any time soon.

As we see the cost of living in our beautiful country escalating, it's increasingly tempting to choose our food purchases based solely on price. It's understandable – we all want value for our money, and feeding a family can be expensive. But there's another way you can get value from what you buy: by buying quality, and having the satisfaction of knowing that the choice you've made rewards others as well as yourself.

In my first cookbook, you may have noticed that there were no pork recipes. I refused to have any, as a statement of my disapproval of the inhumane practices in many of our commercial piggeries. Similarly, I used only sustainable fish in the recipes and directed readers to a website to get the latest information about threatened fish species. For me, it was about drawing a line in the sand and saying, 'This I will do, but this I won't.'

Fortunately, there have been changes for the better since then! Organic, free-range and humanely raised chicken, pork, beef and lamb are now readily available. Supermarkets are increasingly stocking organic fruit and vegetables, and organic produce markets, specialty grocers and delicatessens are popping up everywhere. My husband and I regularly hang out at farmers' markets and organic food markets where you can buy food that is responsibly farmed, uncontaminated by pesticides, seasonal and about as fresh as you can get.

All of the recipes in this book are delicious and nutritious, but you can increase the value and enjoyment you get from cooking and eating them by choosing the ingredients carefully. Not only will you get more for your money nutritionally, but you can bask in the satisfaction of knowing that you've made the best choice for the environment and for the welfare of the animals that ultimately end up on your plate.

Is it more expensive? Not necessarily – in fact, it's often cheaper. The food most definitely lasts a lot longer in my fridge, which is a cost saving for me! But another benefit is the extra value you get for your money by supporting sustainable farming and farmers, and the artisans who produce amazing butters, breads, yoghurts, jams, chutneys, olive oils and cheeses.

These foods also taste better! Their stronger flavours suit the recipes in this book, because you'll notice that the portion sizes aren't big, and may be smaller than you're used to – they're more like the portion sizes that your grandparents would have served. Of course, if you have family members who use lots of energy day-to-day, whether through their work or because they're growing teenagers, then simply increase the portions for them, as your grandparents would have done. After all, whether they're six-foot manual labourers or six-foot growing teenagers, everyone needs to eat healthily, right?

Tuna, chickpea and coriander salad

Tuna and chickpeas make for a satisfying, substantial salad that takes no time to prepare and won't weigh you down during a workday afternoon.

SERVES 2 | PREP 10 minutes | CAL PER SERVE 334

400 g can chickpeas, drained
    and rinsed
180 g can tuna in springwater,
    drained
1 large tomato, coarsely chopped
½ small red onion, thinly sliced

1 bunch coriander, washed
    and coarsely chopped
1 tablespoon extra virgin olive oil
1 tablespoon white-wine vinegar
1 tablespoon lemon juice
freshly ground black pepper

1. Combine the chickpeas, tuna, tomato, onion and coriander in a large bowl. Drizzle with the olive oil, vinegar and lemon juice, and season with pepper. Toss to combine.

TIP: This salad improves after standing for 15 minutes, as the flavours infuse. It's perfect for a lunch box – just make sure to take it out of the fridge 15 minutes before you eat, so it's not too cold.

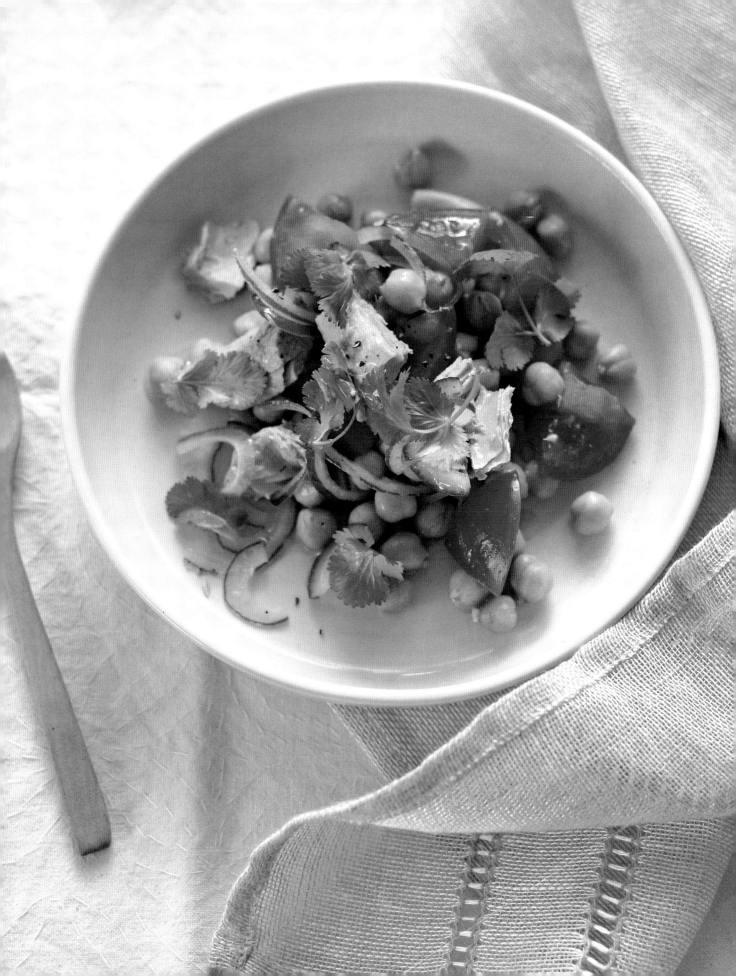

Potato and egg salad with green beans and celery

A new take on an old favourite, salade niçoise – our version is low in calories but big on flavour.

SERVES 2 | **PREP** 15 minutes | **COOK** 15 minutes | **CAL PER SERVE** 308

250 g kipfler potatoes, washed
1½ tablespoons white-wine vinegar
150 g green beans, trimmed
200 g celery, sliced
2 large eggs, hard-boiled and
   quartered
¼ cup pitted kalamata olives, drained
1 tablespoon small sprigs dill

Dressing
1 tablespoon extra virgin olive oil
2 teaspoons Dijon mustard
1 red shallot, finely chopped
freshly ground black pepper

1. Place the potatoes in a medium saucepan, cover with water and bring to the boil. Boil for 12–15 minutes or until tender when pricked with a fork, then drain and slice. Place in a large bowl and drizzle with 2 teaspoons of the vinegar while still warm.

2. Meanwhile, combine the olive oil, mustard, shallot and remaining vinegar in a small bowl. Season with pepper.

3. Bring a small saucepan of salted water to the boil and add the green beans. Cook for 2 minutes until just tender and bright green, then drain and cool in ice-water. Drain again.

4. Add the beans, celery, eggs, olives and dill to the potatoes. Drizzle with the dressing and gently toss to coat.

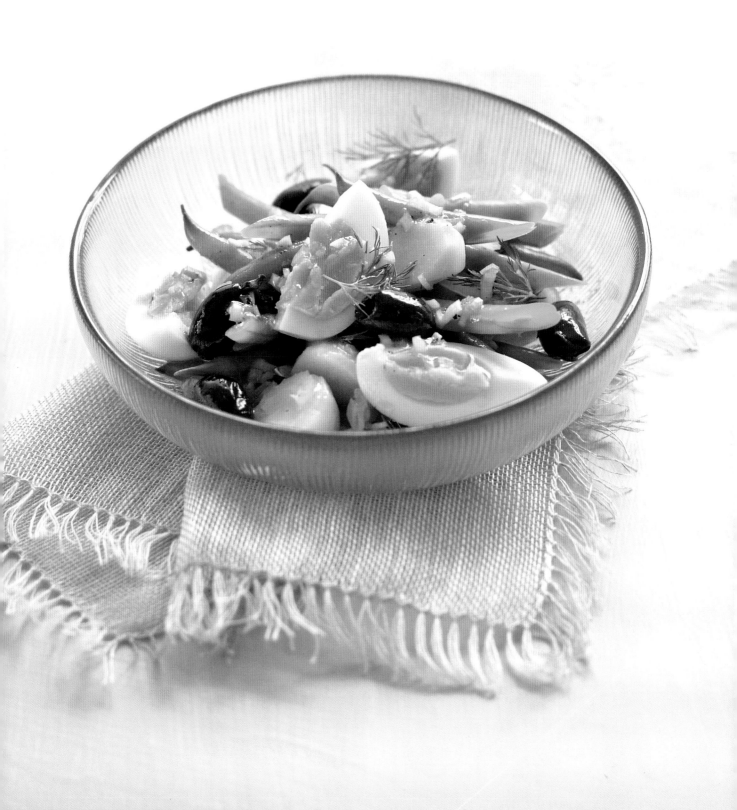

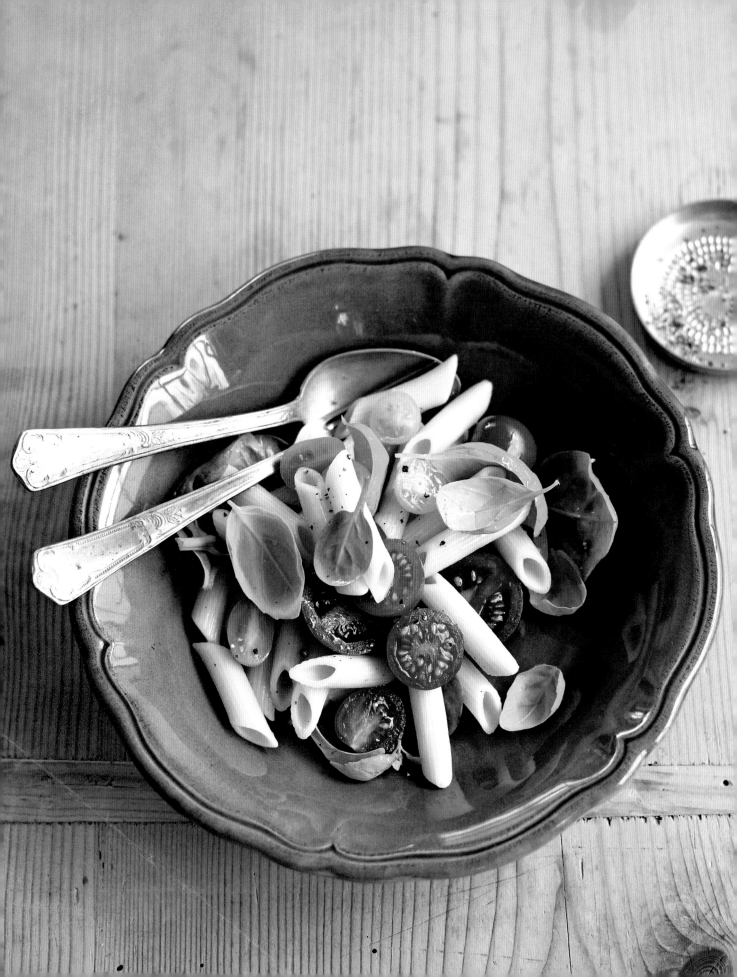

Tomato and basil pasta salad

Pasta? Yep, pasta! Take a look at the portion size and understand that pasta doesn't have to be the enemy!

SERVES 2 | PREP 10 minutes | COOK 15 minutes | CAL PER SERVE 320

125 g dried pasta
250 g mixed baby tomatoes,
    halved
30 g baby spinach

⅓ cup torn basil leaves
1 tablespoon extra virgin olive oil
½ clove garlic, crushed
freshly ground black pepper

1. Cook the pasta in a medium saucepan of boiling salted water according to the packet directions. Drain and cool.

2. Place the pasta, tomatoes, spinach, basil, olive oil and garlic in a large bowl, and season with pepper. Toss to coat.

TIPS: If you feel like a warm pasta dish, you can toss everything together immediately rather than waiting for the pasta to cool.

• Any small pasta, such as penne, orecchiette or dried gnocchi, will be perfect for this recipe.

Lentil, beetroot and feta salad

It's a good idea to wear rubber gloves when dealing with beetroot or you'll have red hands for a while! And if you prefer to keep the feta white for presentation, sprinkle it over the salad after tossing the rest of the ingredients together.

SERVES 2 | **PREP** 15 minutes | **COOK** 45 minutes | **CAL PER SERVE** 333

1 medium beetroot
½ cup dried French-style lentils
40 g low-cal feta, crumbled
200 g celery, sliced on the diagonal
1 red shallot, thinly sliced
¼ cup coarsely chopped parsley

Dressing
1½ tablespoons red-wine vinegar
1 tablespoon extra virgin olive oil
2 teaspoons Dijon mustard
freshly ground black pepper

1. Boil the beetroot in a small saucepan for 40–45 minutes or until tender when pricked with a fork, then drain and stand until cool enough to handle. Peel, discard skin and cut into wedges.

2. Meanwhile, put the lentils into a medium saucepan with 2½ cups of water. Bring to the boil and simmer for 20–25 minutes or until tender, then drain and rinse under cold water.

3. To make the dressing, combine the vinegar, olive oil and mustard in a small bowl and season with pepper.

4. Place the lentils, beetroot, feta, celery, shallot and parsley in a large bowl. Drizzle with the dressing and toss to coat.

TIPS: You can roast the beetroot instead of boiling it if you happen to have the oven on for something else. However, it will take longer – around 40 minutes.

• Canned beetroot can be substituted for fresh if you're pushed for time; you'll need a 225 g can. You can also use canned lentils instead of dried, but the beauty of the French-style ('Puy') lentils is that they keep their shape once cooked, and they're generally not available canned. If you love lentils, try cooking up a big batch and freezing them in portions topped with a little water or cooking liquid.

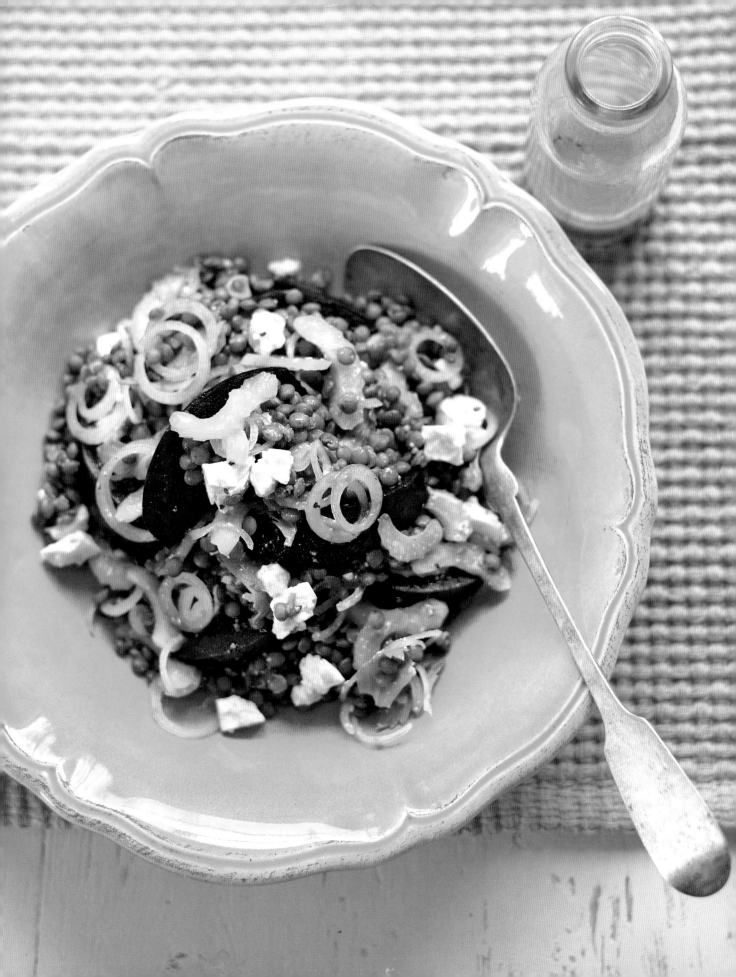

Watercress, fennel and parmesan salad

The garlic gives a great kick in this salad, but you may prefer to omit it if you're making the salad for your lunch box – the flavour does tend to get stronger over time!

SERVES 2 | **PREP** 15 minutes | **COOK** 5 minutes | **CAL PER SERVE** 271

1 bunch watercress, leaves picked
1 fennel bulb, trimmed and
    thinly sliced
⅓ cup shaved parmesan
2 tablespoons pine nuts

Dressing
1 tablespoon extra virgin olive oil
2 teaspoons lemon juice
2 anchovies, finely chopped
½ clove garlic, crushed
freshly ground black pepper

1. Place the watercress, fennel and half the parmesan in a salad bowl.

2. To make the dressing, put the olive oil, lemon juice, anchovies and garlic in a small bowl or empty jam jar. Season with freshly ground black pepper and stir (or shake) vigorously.

3. Toast the pine nuts in a small frying pan on medium heat for 2–3 minutes until golden.

4. Drizzle the dressing over the salad and toss to coat, then sprinkle with the pine nuts and the remaining parmesan.

TIP: It's important to dress the salad at the last moment to prevent the watercress from wilting, so if you're making this for your lunch box, take the dressing in a separate container.

White bean, tomato and basil salad

A fresh, filling salad that's great for lunch or to serve at a barbecue with the lamb from the Char-grilled lamb and vegetable salad (page 110).

SERVES 2 | PREP 15 minutes | CAL PER SERVE 300

400 g can cannellini beans, drained
   and rinsed
250 g cherry tomatoes, halved
1 fennel bulb, trimmed and
   thinly sliced
½ bunch basil, leaves torn
¼ cup pitted kalamata olives in brine,
   drained and coarsely chopped
freshly ground black pepper

Dressing
1 tablespoon extra virgin olive oil
1 tablespoon white balsamic vinegar

1. Combine the beans, tomatoes, fennel, basil and olives in a salad bowl. To make the dressing, combine the olive oil and vinegar in a glass jar and shake to mix.

2. Drizzle the dressing over the salad, season with freshly ground black pepper and toss to coat. Serve immediately.

TIPS: This is also delicious with a 400 g can of chickpeas (288 cal per serve) instead of cannellini beans.

• Cooking your own pulses from dried is a great idea – they taste better, contain less salt and it's much cheaper! Cook up a big batch and freeze the leftovers in individual portions, with a little cooking liquid so they won't dry out. (About 110 g of dried beans makes 260 g cooked – which is the net weight of a 400 g can.)

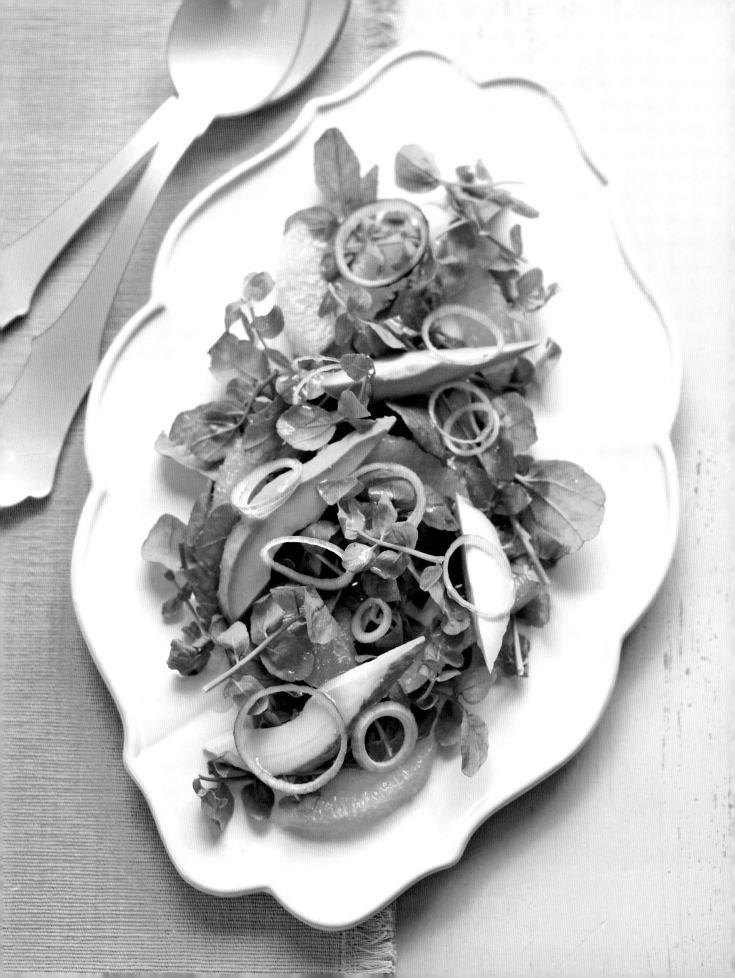

Orange and watercress salad

Clean, fresh flavours, creamy avocado and a kick of sweetness
from the oranges – it's a total winner.

SERVES 2 | PREP 15 minutes | CAL PER SERVE 325

2 oranges
1 medium avocado, sliced
1 bunch watercress, leaves picked
¼ red onion, thinly sliced

1 tablespoon extra virgin olive oil
2 teaspoons sherry vinegar
freshly ground black pepper

1. Peel the oranges and cut away the segments
over a bowl to catch the juice as well.
Add the remaining ingredients to the bowl,
season with pepper and gently toss to coat.

TIP: This salad tastes best if left to stand
for 15 minutes before serving.

Tandoori chicken with carrot salad

Spices are the difference between an average meal and a fantastic one, in my opinion. Tandoori seasoning is so great for chicken, and the black mustard seeds add crunch and heat to the carrot salad.

SERVES 2 | **PREP** 15 minutes | **COOK** 20 minutes | **CAL PER SERVE** 319

220 g chicken breast fillets
1 tablespoon tandoori seasoning
cooking oil spray

Indian grated carrot salad
2 tablespoons shredded coconut
2 teaspoons vegetable oil

¼ teaspoon black mustard seeds
8 fresh curry leaves
½ small red onion, finely chopped
½ long green chilli, finely chopped
300 g carrots, grated
freshly ground black pepper
1 tablespoon sultanas

1. For the salad, tip the coconut into a small bowl and cover with ¼ cup of boiling water. Stand for 10 minutes, then drain.

2. Meanwhile, heat the oil in a large saucepan on high. Add the mustard seeds and cook for 1 minute until they crackle, then add the curry leaves, onion and chilli and cook, stirring, for 5 minutes until the onion is soft. Add the coconut and cook for another minute. Stir in the carrot and season to taste, then reduce the heat to low and cook, covered, for 4 minutes until the carrot is just tender. Stir through the sultanas.

3. Sprinkle the chicken fillets with the tandoori seasoning. Lightly spray a char-grill with oil and heat on medium–high, then grill the chicken for 4–5 minutes each side or until just cooked through.

4. Serve the chicken thickly sliced with the grated carrot salad.

TIP: This South Indian salad is also terrific with other vegetables, like green beans, cauliflower and zucchini.

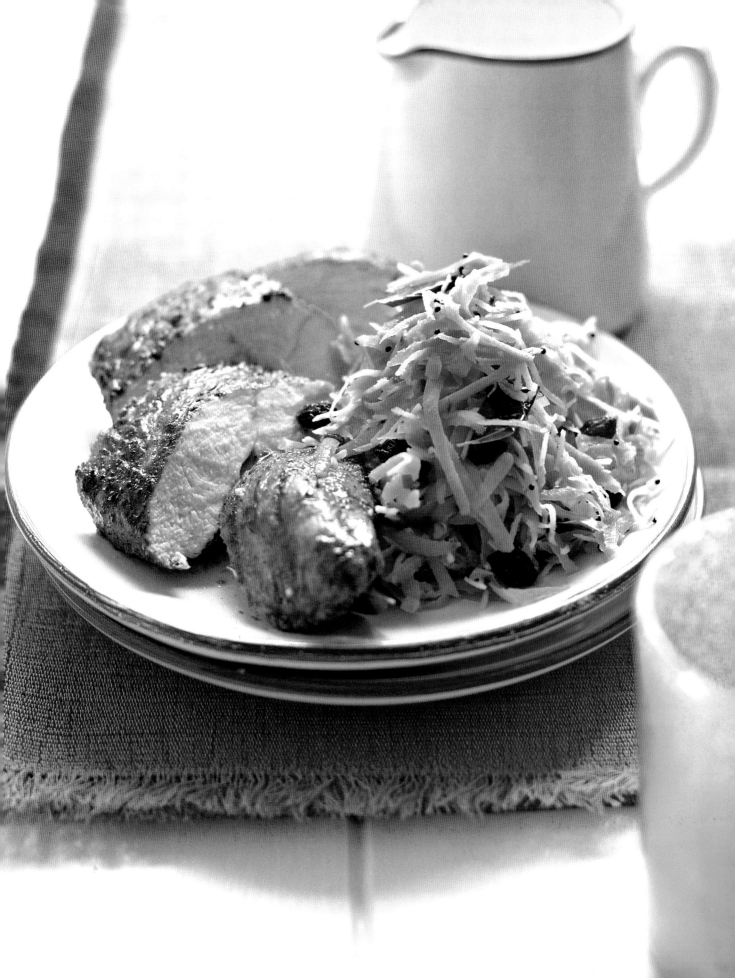

Vietnamese beef salad

You'll love this crisp, refreshing salad. Don't be afraid of the fish sauce: it's pungent by itself, but with the lemongrass and garlic it adds a subtle savouriness that you can't get any other way.

SERVES 2 | **PREP** 15 minutes | **COOK** 10 minutes | **CAL PER SERVE** 339

1 lemongrass stalk, finely chopped
2 cloves garlic, crushed
1 tablespoon fish sauce
125 g beef rump steak, trimmed
 of fat and thinly sliced
100 g rice vermicelli noodles
cooking oil spray

1 carrot, grated
½ Lebanese cucumber,
 chopped into thin strips
⅛ iceberg lettuce, shredded
1 bunch mint, leaves picked
2 tablespoons pre-prepared
 Vietnamese dipping sauce

1. Place the lemongrass, garlic and fish sauce in a small food processor and process until very finely chopped. Reserve half of the mixture; combine the rest with the beef in a medium bowl and toss to coat.

2. Cook the vermicelli noodles according to the packet directions. Drain.

3. Lightly spray a wok with oil, heat on medium–high and stir-fry the reserved lemongrass mixture until fragrant. Spoon it over the noodles and toss to coat.

4. Divide the noodles between two large serving bowls and arrange the carrot, cucumber, lettuce and mint in each bowl.

5. Lightly spray the wok with oil again and heat on high. Stir-fry the beef for 1–2 minutes or until browned but still rare, then divide between the serving bowls, drizzle with dipping sauce and serve immediately.

TIP: This salad is great made in advance for your lunch box.

Snacks

Stick to wholefoods and eat small portions no more than 100 to 150 calories, and you can eat snacks without blowing your weight-loss or maintenance efforts. Here are a few ideas:

- A medium banana or apple, a cup of strawberries or 20 grapes = around 75 cal
- 1½ cups of unsalted edamame in their pods = 100 cal
- 2 cups of air-popped popcorn without salt or butter = 60 cal
- A tub of low-cal yoghurt = 81 cal
- 1 cup of low-cal hot chocolate and 10 fresh cherries = 114 cal
- 3 thick slices of tomato, topped with a slice of bocconcini and a large basil leaf = around 71 cal
- 2 celery stalks dipped into 2 tablespoons of hummus = 100 cal
- 2 large iceberg lettuce leaves filled with ½ cup of leftover cooked chicken and 1 tablespoon of tomato salsa = 150 cal
- 1 cup of frozen mixed berries, 3 tablespoons of low-cal yoghurt and 4 ice cubes blended together into a frappe = 140 cal
- 1 slice of low-GI fruit bread, fresh or toasted, spread with low-cal cream cheese = around 104 cal

Of course, you don't have to eat snacks if you don't feel the need: just have slightly larger meals instead to make up your daily calorie quota. I had a bit of a wake-up call about this while I was away on holiday recently. I realised that I didn't eat one snack, because we were too busy walking and discovering things. I really think we put too much importance on snacks. Yes, sometimes we actually need them, but I wonder whether a lot of the time we eat them purely out of habit or boredom.

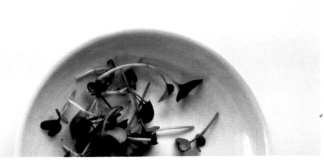

Vegetable and barley soup

Soup is a great basic for winter lunches. In this recipe, the pearl barley
and lentils make for a warming, substantial meal.

SERVES 4 | PREP 10 minutes | COOK 50 minutes | CAL PER SERVE 242

1 tablespoon olive oil
1 brown onion, diced
3 stalks celery, trimmed and sliced
2 cloves garlic, crushed
1 teaspoon ground turmeric
6 cups good-quality vegetable stock

½ cup pearl barley
1 large carrot, halved and sliced
½ cup red lentils, rinsed and drained
200 g green beans, trimmed and
   cut into 3 cm pieces
½ cup coriander leaves

1. Heat the olive oil in a large saucepan on
   medium–high. Cook the onion, celery and
   garlic for 5 minutes until softened, then stir
   in the turmeric and cook until fragrant.

2. Add the stock and barley, bring to the
   boil and simmer, covered, for 30 minutes.
   Stir in the carrot and lentils and simmer,
   covered, for 5 minutes. Add the beans and
   simmer for 10 minutes until the vegetables,
   barley and lentils are tender.

3. Serve sprinkled with coriander.

TIP: This recipe makes 8 cups (2 litres).

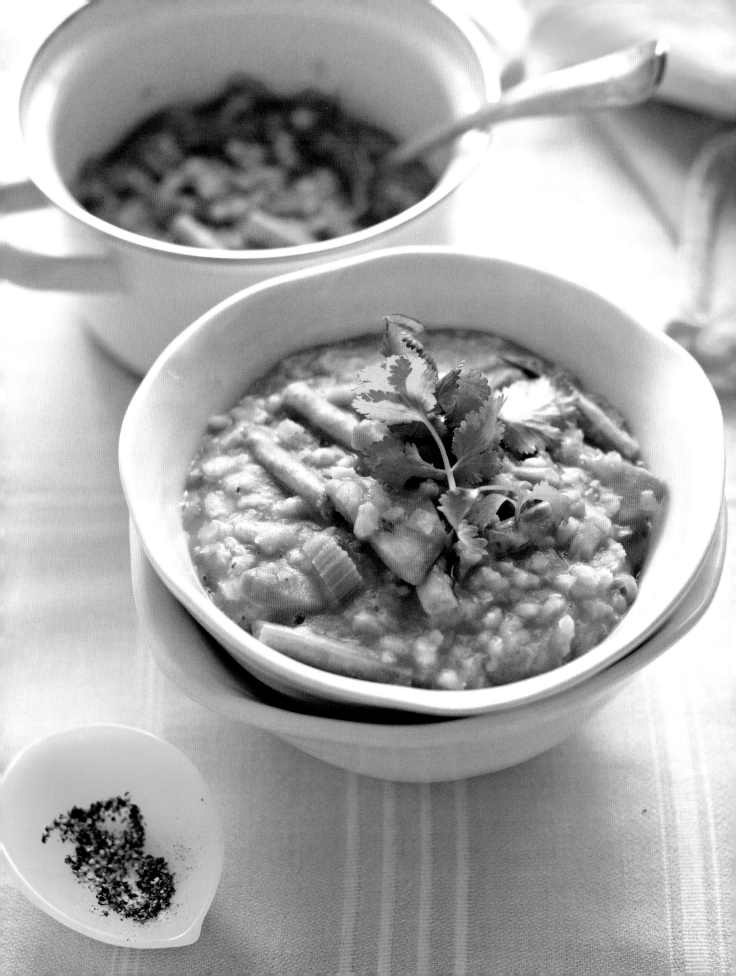

Gazpacho

A Spanish classic that knocks it out of the park for lunch or supper on hot summer days. This also makes an impressive dinner party starter served in tiny cups with a garnish of ice cubes and mint.

SERVES 4 | PREP 15 minutes | COOK 5 minutes | CHILL 2 hours | CAL PER SERVE 252

1.2 kg ripe tomatoes
1 long cucumber, chopped
½ green capsicum, peeled
½ red capsicum, peeled
1 brown onion, chopped
1 clove garlic
2 tablespoons sherry vinegar
2 tablespoons extra virgin olive oil
freshly ground black pepper

Topping
2 eggs, hard-boiled and diced
½ green capsicum, diced
½ red capsicum, diced
40 g wholegrain bread,
   toasted and diced

1. Make a small cut at the base of each tomato. Bring a large saucepan of water to the boil, add the tomatoes and boil for 15–20 seconds or until the skins tear. Remove immediately with a slotted spoon and place in ice-water until cold, then drain. Peel and discard the skins and seeds.

2. Combine the peeled tomatoes, cucumber, capsicum, onion and garlic in a large food processor or blender and process until smooth. Stir in the vinegar and olive oil and season with pepper. Refrigerate the soup for 2 hours or until well chilled.

3. To make the topping, combine all the ingredients and divide the mixture between small serving bowls so people can help themselves.

TIPS: You can use a standard vegetable peeler to peel the capsicum.

• This recipe makes 8 cups (2 litres). The soup is quite thick: if you prefer it thinner, just add a little water.

• If you haven't got time to chill the soup, serve it with ice cubes.

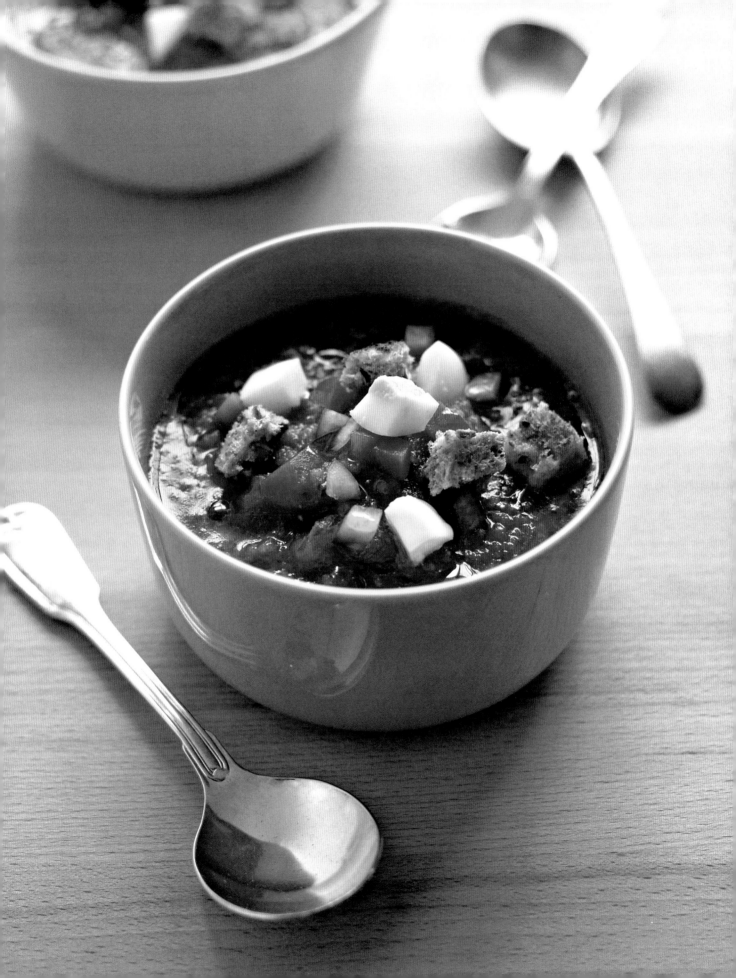

Lebanese lentil soup

Packed with nutrients from the silverbeet, with rice and lentils adding a nutty heft – and you won't believe how deliciously tangy the lemon juice makes this soup.

SERVES 5 | **PREP** 15 minutes | **COOK** 1 hour 20 minutes | **CAL PER SERVE** 305

1½ cups brown lentils
1 tablespoon olive oil
2 brown onions, sliced
½ cup brown medium-grain rice

6 silverbeet leaves, shredded
1½ tablespoons lemon juice
freshly ground black pepper

1. Place the lentils and 4 cups of water in a large saucepan, and bring to the boil. Simmer, covered, for 40 minutes or until the lentils are tender, then coarsely mash them with a potato masher.

2. Meanwhile, heat the olive oil in a large frying pan on high and cook the onion, stirring, for 8 minutes or until golden.

3. Stir the rice, half the onion and 5 cups of water through the lentils. Bring to the boil, then cover and simmer for 40 minutes or until the rice is tender. Stir in the shredded silverbeet and simmer for another minute, then stir in the lemon juice and season with freshly ground black pepper.

4. Serve garnished with the remaining onion.

TIPS: This recipe makes about 9 cups of soup, but you may need to add more water to get the consistency you like, as the lentils and rice will keep soaking up the liquid.

• If you divide the soup into 6 serves, it's 247 cal per serve.

Zucchini and curry soup

In early autumn, this soup is a great way to use up a glut of
zucchini from your garden. Herbs and spices add punch.

SERVES 6 | PREP 20 minutes | COOK 20 minutes | CAL PER SERVE 280

2 tablespoons olive oil
2 kg zucchini, trimmed and chopped
10 spring onions, coarsely chopped
1 tablespoon mild curry powder

2 teaspoons ground cumin
4 cups good-quality chicken stock
6 small pieces naan
1 bunch chives, finely chopped

1. Heat the olive oil in a large saucepan on
   medium, then stir in the zucchini
   and spring onion. Reduce the heat to
   low and cook, covered, for 12 minutes
   until tender, stirring occasionally.

2. Add the spices and cook for a further
   2 minutes, stirring. Stir in the stock
   and 2 cups of water and cook for another
   minute. Allow the soup to cool slightly and
   then puree, in batches, in a food processor
   or blender. Return it to the saucepan and
   reheat gently. Meanwhile, toast the naan.

3. Serve sprinkled with chives, with a piece
   of warm naan per person.

TIP: This recipe makes about 12 cups.

Chicken and udon noodle soup

Noodles, chicken, ginger, greens and coriander – you just can't ask for better than this clean-tasting, satisfying soup. Love it!

SERVES 2 | PREP 10 minutes | COOK 25 minutes | CAL PER SERVE 275

4 spring onions
4 cups good-quality chicken stock
45 g ginger, peeled and sliced
2 star anise
200 g chicken breast, skin off

1 bunch baby bok choy,
 washed and leaves separated
200 g udon noodles
1 tablespoon low-salt soy sauce
1 cup coriander leaves

1. Finely slice one of the spring onions on the diagonal and reserve. Coarsely chop the remainder.

2. Combine the stock, ginger, star anise and coarsely chopped spring onion with 2 cups of water in a medium saucepan. Bring to the boil, then reduce the heat and simmer, covered, for 10 minutes. Add the chicken and simmer for 8 minutes or until just cooked through, then remove with a slotted spoon and stand to cool slightly. Slice or shred the chicken once it's cool enough to handle.

3. Strain the broth into a large bowl and discard the ginger, star anise and spring onion. Return the liquid to the pan, bring to a simmer and add the bok choy, noodles and soy sauce. Stir until the leaves have wilted and the noodles have softened, then stir through the chicken, coriander and reserved spring onion to serve.

TIP: If you're buying the chicken stock, look out for a salt-reduced variety. But it's easy to make your own – and it will taste 100 times better and not be too salty or fatty. Here's how:

Buy a chicken carcass from your butcher, trim it of all fat and place it in a large saucepan with a chopped carrot, a celery stalk, an onion, a couple of cloves of garlic, a bay leaf and some black peppercorns. Add water to cover the chicken, and bring to the boil. Simmer gently for 30 minutes, skimming regularly, then strain the stock into a large bowl and discard the carcass and vegetables. Refrigerate until the fat has set (around 8–12 hours), so it's easier to scoop it away and discard it.

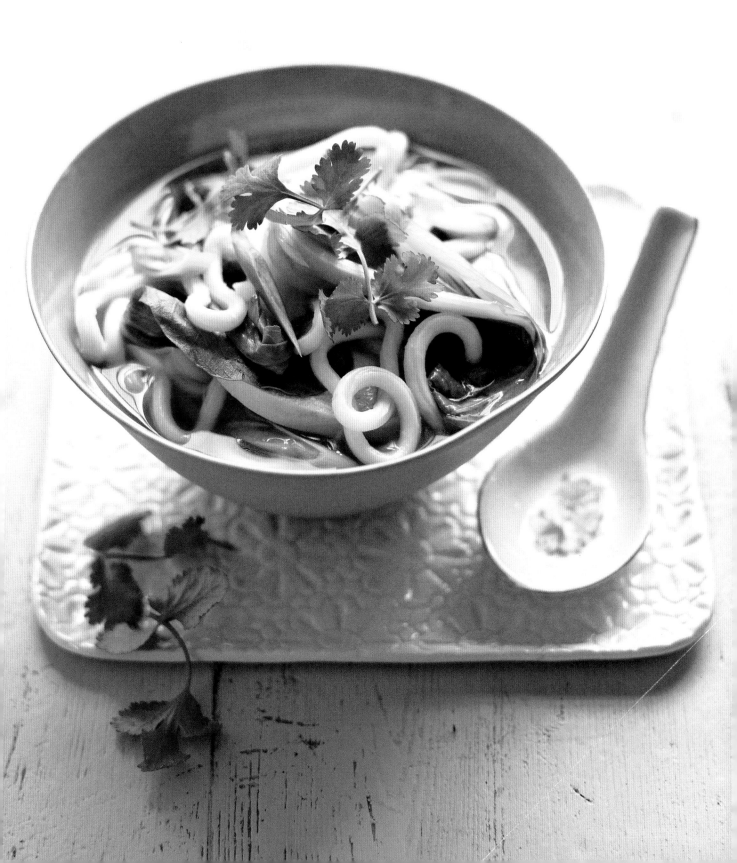

Lamb and white bean soup with spinach

Another knockout soup that ticks all the boxes with vegetables, beans and spinach. The rich, nourishing combo of lamb shanks and red wine is unbeatable.

SERVES 4 | PREP 20 minutes | COOK 2 hours | CAL PER SERVE 241

olive oil spray
2 lamb shanks, trimmed of fat
1 teaspoon olive oil
1 brown onion, diced
1 carrot, diced
3 cloves garlic, sliced

1 cup red wine
2 tablespoons tomato paste
2 × 400 g cans butter beans,
   drained and rinsed
100 g baby spinach

1. Lightly spray a large saucepan with olive oil and heat on medium–high. Cook the lamb shanks, turning, for 5 minutes or until browned all over. Remove them from the pan and discard any juices.

2. Heat the olive oil in the same pan over medium heat, and cook the onion, carrot and garlic, stirring, for 5 minutes until softened. Return the shanks to the pan, add the wine and tomato paste, and bring to the boil. Add 6 cups of water and bring to the boil again, then reduce the heat and simmer, covered, for 1½ hours until the lamb is tender and the meat falls off the bone. Remove the shanks with a slotted spoon.

3. Stir in the beans and simmer for 10 minutes. Meanwhile, shred the lamb meat from the bone, discard the bone and return the meat to the pan. Simmer until heated through, stir in the spinach and serve.

TIPS: This recipe makes 8 cups (2 litres).

• Accompanying the soup with 2 slices of toasted wholemeal bread per person increases the calories to 352 cal per serve.

Clint from Ipswich, 39

Starting weight: 110 kg

At the time of writing: 84 kg

Before, I simply felt unwell. I was constantly bloated and often felt sick after meals. The day I chose to make a change was the day my belt no longer fitted and I realised I was considering buying a bigger one.

My wife and children and I had take-out for dinner four nights a week. We knew the menus so well that we didn't have to think about what to order. It was a 'drive in, drive out' mentality: we'd convinced ourselves it was quicker and cheaper. In the back of my mind I thought that healthy food was too expensive, even though I was easily spending $30 to $40 a night on take-out!

What hit me hard was what I was doing to my kids – I'd trained them to think that eating take-out regularly was the norm. My wife and I had to stay united and lead by example to wean them off eating it. It was tough at first, but now they're much better. We allow them to have the occasional take-out meal as a treat, and now they see it as that.

I loved the convenience factor of Michelle's shopping lists. We simply walked through the shopping aisles and purchased what was on the list, no deviation required. It was also convenient that we had the food at home ready to prepare. Michelle's meals took us no time to put together and literally within a week I started to lose weight and feel so much better about myself.

Mushroom and silverbeet lasagne

Lasagne is a family favourite everywhere. We've swapped the bolognese for silverbeet and a garlicky mushroom mix, to make a lighter and extra-nutritious version that still tastes wonderful.

SERVES 6 | **PREP** 30 minutes | **COOK** 1 hour 30 minutes | **CAL PER SERVE** 290

olive oil spray
1 brown onion, diced
400 g mushrooms, coarsely
   chopped or sliced
3 cloves garlic, crushed
1 tablespoon finely chopped
   fresh thyme
freshly ground black pepper
600 g silverbeet, trimmed and
   washed, stems thinly sliced
   and leaves coarsely chopped

400 g can diced tomatoes
2½ tablespoons cornflour
2½ cups low-fat milk
10 (15 cm × 8 cm) sheets dried lasagne
¾ cup low-fat grated mozzarella
½ cup finely grated parmesan
100 g mesclun salad mix, to serve

1. Preheat your oven to 180°C.

2. Lightly spray a deep frying pan with olive oil and heat on medium–high. Add the onion and cook, stirring, for 5 minutes until softened. Add the mushrooms, garlic and thyme and cook, stirring occasionally, for 8 minutes or until golden and the moisture has evaporated. Season with pepper and remove the vegetables from the pan.

3. Heat the same pan on high. Add the silverbeet and cook, stirring occasionally, until the leaves are wilted and the moisture has evaporated. Stir in the tomatoes and bring to the boil, then simmer for 10 minutes or until the sauce thickens. Season with pepper.

4. Meanwhile, combine the cornflour and ¼ cup of the milk in a jug. Pour the remaining milk into a saucepan and bring to the boil on high, then whisk in the cornflour mixture and cook, stirring, for 2–3 minutes until the sauce boils and thickens. Season well with pepper.

5. Lightly spray an 8-cup ovenproof dish with olive oil. Cover the base of the dish with a little silverbeet mixture and top with lasagne sheets. Combine the cheeses. Cover the sheets with half of the silverbeet mixture and then half of the mushroom mix, drizzle over a third of the white sauce and sprinkle with a third of the mixed cheeses. Add another layer of lasagne sheets and repeat the filling layers. Finish with a final layer of pasta sheets and the remaining third of the white sauce and cheese, and bake for 1 hour until the pasta is tender and the top is golden.

6. Serve with the mesclun.

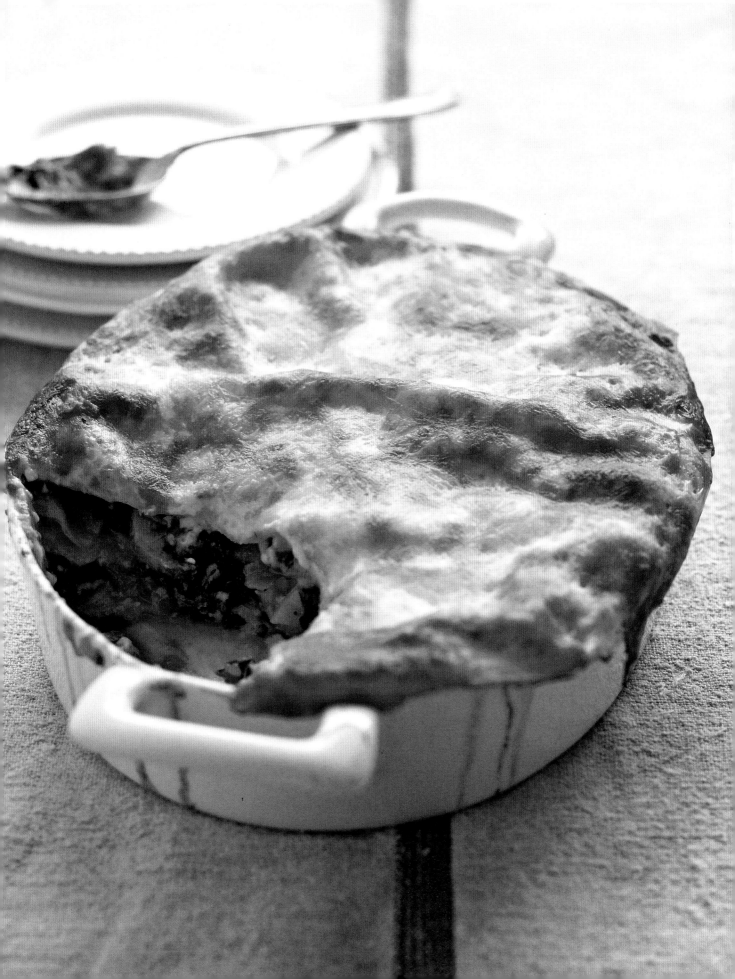

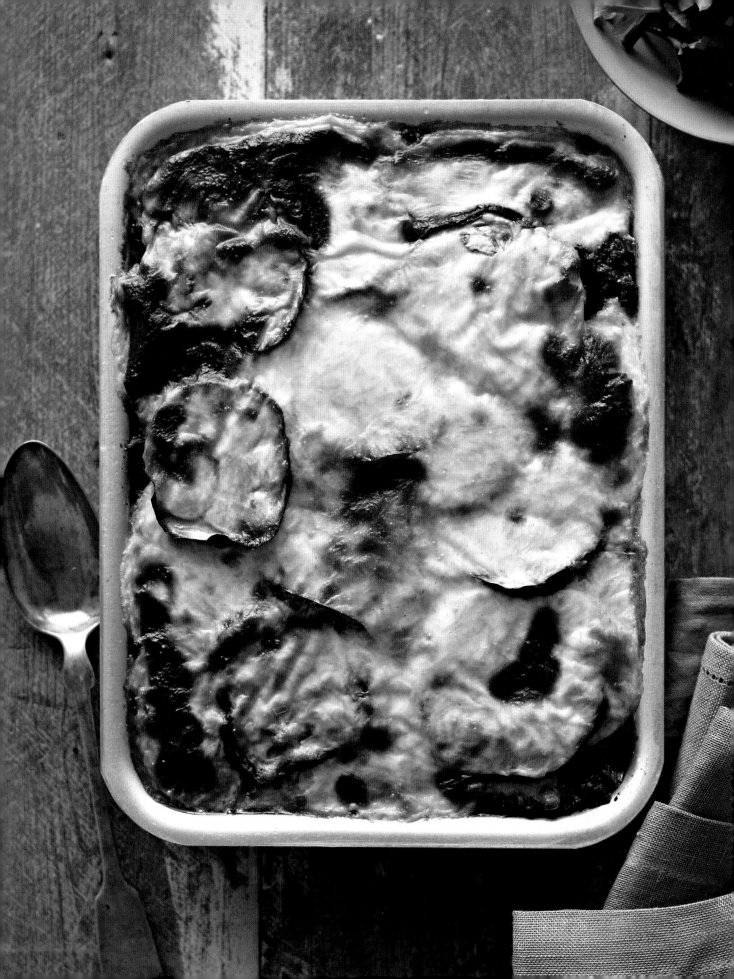

Moussaka

You can freeze portions of this moussaka in airtight containers –
it makes a fantastic weeknight standby.

SERVES 6 | **PREP** 20 minutes | **COOK** 1 hour 20 minutes | **CAL PER SERVE** 243

1 kg eggplant, trimmed
    and thickly sliced
olive oil spray
1 brown onion, finely chopped
2 cloves garlic, crushed
400 g lean lamb mince
400 g can diced tomatoes
2 teaspoons dried oregano

½ teaspoon ground cinnamon
½ teaspoon ground allspice
freshly ground black pepper
1½ tablespoons cornflour
1½ cups low-cal milk
¾ cup grated parmesan
1 egg yolk
100 g mixed leaves, to serve

1. Preheat your oven to 180°C.

2. Bring some water to the boil in a saucepan with a steamer insert, and steam the eggplant for 10 minutes until very soft. Drain on paper towel.

3. Meanwhile, lightly spray a large frying pan with olive oil and heat on medium. Cook the onion and garlic, stirring, for 5 minutes until softened. Increase the heat to high and add the mince. Cook for 5 minutes, breaking up any lumps with a spoon, until brown and the liquid has evaporated. Add the tomatoes, oregano and spices, and season with pepper. Simmer, stirring occasionally, for 10 minutes.

4. Combine the cornflour and ¼ cup of the milk in a jug. Pour the remaining milk into a saucepan and bring to the boil on high, then whisk in the cornflour mixture. Cook, stirring, for 2–3 minutes until the sauce boils and thickens. Remove from the heat and whisk in the parmesan and egg yolk.

5. Line the base of an 8-cup ovenproof dish with a third of the steamed eggplant and top with half of the lamb mixture. Repeat the layers, then top with the remaining eggplant and spoon over the white sauce. Bake the moussaka for 45 minutes until golden. Stand for 10 minutes.

6. Serve hot or at room temperature with the mixed leaves.

Chickpea and vegetable Madras curry

Plain yoghurt makes this curry a creamy, satisfying way to sneak in plenty of veggies.

SERVES 4 | **PREP** 20 minutes | **COOK** 40 minutes | **CAL PER SERVE** 278

1 tablespoon vegetable oil
2 brown onions, cut into wedges
4 cloves garlic, crushed
1 tablespoon grated ginger
2 tablespoons Madras curry paste
1 large tomato, diced
½ cup plain low-cal yoghurt

400 g can chickpeas, drained
  and rinsed
500 g cauliflower, broken into florets
1 large red capsicum, cut into chunks
200 g green beans, trimmed
  and halved
½ cup coriander leaves

1. Heat the oil in a large saucepan on medium–high and cook the onion, stirring, for 10 minutes or until well browned and softened. Stir in the garlic, ginger and curry paste and cook for 1 minute. Turn the heat down to medium, add the tomato and cook for 1–2 minutes, stirring, until it starts to break down.

2. Stir in the yoghurt well. Add the chickpeas, cauliflower and capsicum and simmer, covered, for 15 minutes, then stir in the beans, cover again, and simmer for another 10 minutes until the vegetables are tender.

3. Serve sprinkled with coriander.

TIP: Curry pastes are quite oily, so make sure you give the Madras paste a good stir before measuring out the 2 tablespoons.

Greek lamb shanks with lentils

With easy prep but long, slow cooking, these shanks are lovely for a weekend lunch with friends. Definitely worth the wait!

SERVES 4 | **PREP** 15 minutes | **COOK** 2 hours 15 minutes | **CAL PER SERVE** 355

olive oil spray
4 frenched lamb shanks,
   trimmed of fat
1 large brown onion, finely chopped
2 stalks celery, diced
3 large carrots, cut into large chunks

1 bay leaf
½ cup brown lentils, drained
   and rinsed
1 tablespoon lemon juice
2 tablespoons coarsely
   chopped parsley

1. Lightly spray a large heavy-based saucepan with olive oil and heat on medium–high. Add the lamb and cook until browned all over. Remove from the pan.

2. Cook the onion, celery, carrot and bay leaf, stirring, for about 5 minutes or until softened. Then return the lamb to the pan with 4 cups of water, bring it to the boil and simmer, covered, for 1 hour. Turn the shanks halfway through.

3. Stir in the lentils and simmer, covered, for another hour until the lamb and lentils are tender.

4. Stir in the lemon juice and serve the dish sprinkled with parsley.

Fish stew

This stew has a beautiful, simple fish flavour, but you could also add a bay leaf – or a finely chopped chilli if you like things hot.

SERVES 4 | **PREP** 15 minutes | **COOK** 1 hour | **CAL PER SERVE** 344

1 tablespoon olive oil
2 large brown onions, thickly sliced
2 large red capsicums, sliced into thick rings
1 ripe tomato, diced
400 g large potatoes, skin on, thickly sliced

500 g monkfish fillets, skin off and deboned
½ cup dry white wine
freshly ground black pepper
2 tablespoons flat-leaf parsley leaves

1. Add the olive oil to a large, heavy-based casserole dish. In the dish, layer the onion, capsicum, tomato, potato and fish. Pour over the wine and ¼ cup of water and season.

2. Cover and cook on medium for 45–60 minutes until the vegetables are tender and the fish is just cooked through. Serve sprinkled with parsley.

TIPS: Angelfish fillets or a mix of several thick fish fillets will also work in this dish if you can't find monkfish.

• The trick with this stew is to keep it covered, so that all the steam stays inside and the fish remains moist. It should flake easily with a fork when it's cooked.

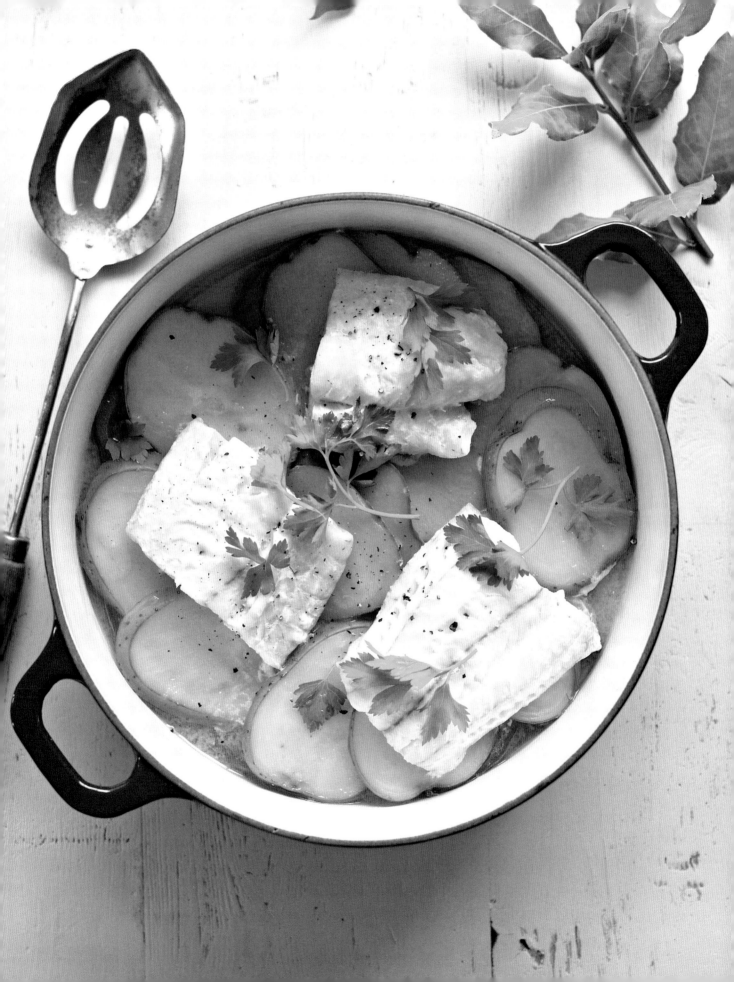

Osso buco with polenta

Osso buco and polenta? It spells winter weekend to me.
Don't skip the gremolata!

SERVES 6 | **PREP** 20 minutes | **COOK** 1 hour 45 minutes | **CAL PER SERVE** 380

¼ cup plain flour
freshly ground black pepper
1 kg veal osso buco pieces
1 tablespoon olive oil
2 brown onions, diced
2 large carrots, cut into large chunks
1 clove garlic, chopped
2 anchovies, chopped
½ cup dry white wine
1 cup good-quality beef stock
2 tablespoons tomato paste

Gremolata
¼ cup chopped parsley
2 cloves garlic, finely chopped
2 tablespoons finely grated lemon zest

Polenta
1 cup polenta
½ cup finely grated parmesan

1. Preheat your oven to 180°C.

2. Pour the flour onto a plate and season it with freshly ground black pepper. Add the veal and turn to coat it with flour, shaking off any excess.

3. Heat the olive oil in a large flameproof casserole dish on medium–high, and cook the veal in batches for 2–3 minutes a side, until well browned. Add the onion and carrot and cook until softened, then stir in the garlic and the anchovy and cook until fragrant. Add the wine, and cook for 3–5 minutes until it evaporates.

4. Combine the stock and tomato paste in a small bowl, then add the mixture to the dish and bring it to the boil. Cover the dish and put it in the oven to cook for 1½ hours, until the meat is very tender.

5. To make the gremolata, combine all the ingredients in a small bowl.

6. To make the polenta, pour 5 cups of water into a large saucepan and bring it to the boil on high. Reduce the heat to medium and sprinkle in the polenta in a slow stream, stirring constantly. Reduce the heat to low and cook for 6 minutes, stirring frequently, until the polenta is tender. Stand uncovered for 10 minutes, before stirring in the parmesan.

7. Serve the osso buco on a bed of polenta and sprinkle the meat with the gremolata.

Chicken meatloaf

This tangy, layered meatloaf is super-versatile: attractive enough in its silverbeet wrapping for a picnic or lunch with friends, but also a great basic for the lunch box or as a weeknight supper with a green salad.

SERVES 8 | **PREP** 30 minutes | **COOK** 1 hour 15 minutes
COOL 1 hour | **CHILL** 4 hours | **CAL PER SERVE** 213

olive oil spray
6 silverbeet leaves, trimmed
600 g chicken breast fillets, skin off
600 g chicken thigh fillets, skin off
3 teaspoons Dijon mustard

3 teaspoons finely chopped
  fresh tarragon
1 teaspoon lemon zest
freshly ground black pepper
1 bunch asparagus, trimmed

1. Preheat your oven to 200°C. Lightly spray a loaf pan (23 cm × 10 cm × 7.5 cm high) with olive oil, then line the base and the two long sides with baking paper, extending the paper 5 cm above both sides.

2. Bring a large saucepan of water to the boil, add the silverbeet leaves and cook until wilted. Put the leaves immediately into a bowl of ice-water until cool, then drain on paper towel.

3. Line the base and the sides of the pan with the silverbeet, slightly overlapping the leaves and allowing an overhang on the long sides of the pan.

4. Chop the chicken into cubes, then put half of it into a food processor and process until finely minced. In a large bowl, combine the mince with the remaining chopped chicken and the mustard, tarragon and lemon zest. Season. Place a third of the mixture into the pan and add half the asparagus, pushing it slightly into the chicken mixture.

5. Repeat the layers with another third of the chicken mixture and the rest of the asparagus. Top with the remaining chicken mixture, press down, and fold the silverbeet over the top to cover the meatloaf. Fold over the extending baking paper, too, and cover the pan tightly with foil.

6. Place the pan in a large roasting dish and add enough boiling water to come halfway up the sides of the pan. Bake for 1 hour 15 minutes, remove from the oven and carefully drain the juices from the pan. Stand until cool.

7. Weigh the meatloaf down with heavy cans and refrigerate for at least 4 hours. Then turn it onto a board lined with paper towel and slice it into 8 portions.

TIP: If you're serving 6, this has 284 cal per serve.

Roasted chicken with beetroot and orange salad

You can't go past a roast chicken for pure comfort food. The beetroot and orange salad is a sweet, earthy accompaniment.

SERVES 6 | **PREP** 20 minutes | **COOK** 1 hour | **CAL PER SERVE** 355

1.6 kg whole chicken,
   trimmed and washed
half a lemon
freshly ground black pepper
olive oil spray

Roasted beetroot and orange salad
1 kg beetroot
2 oranges, segmented, juice reserved
1 bunch mint, leaves picked
1 tablespoon extra virgin olive oil

1. Preheat your oven to 200°C.

2. Pat the chicken dry with some paper towel. Squeeze some lemon juice into the chicken cavity, then place the lemon half inside. Season the cavity with pepper and truss the chicken with kitchen string.

3. Place the trussed chicken onto a wire rack on a roasting tray, spray lightly with olive oil and season with pepper. Roast for 1 hour, basting regularly, until the chicken juices run clear when you pierce the thickest part with a skewer. Stand, loosely covered, for 5 minutes before carving and removing the skin.

4. Meanwhile, to make the salad, line a roasting dish with foil, place the beetroot on top and cover with more foil. Roast for 1 hour until tender. When the beetroot is cool enough to handle, slip off and discard the skins and chop into wedges. In a large bowl, combine the wedges with the orange segments and juice, mint leaves and olive oil, then season with pepper and toss to coat.

5. Serve the chicken without the skin and with the salad.

TIPS: Use rubber gloves when handling beetroot, to avoid getting purple stains on your hands.

• If your oven is big enough, put the chicken and the beetroot on the same shelf. If not, you can use different shelves but you'll need to set your oven to 180°C fan-forced, so that the heat circulates and everything cooks evenly.

• Leaving the chicken skin on makes this 432 cal per serve!

• The salad on its own is only 105 cal per serve.

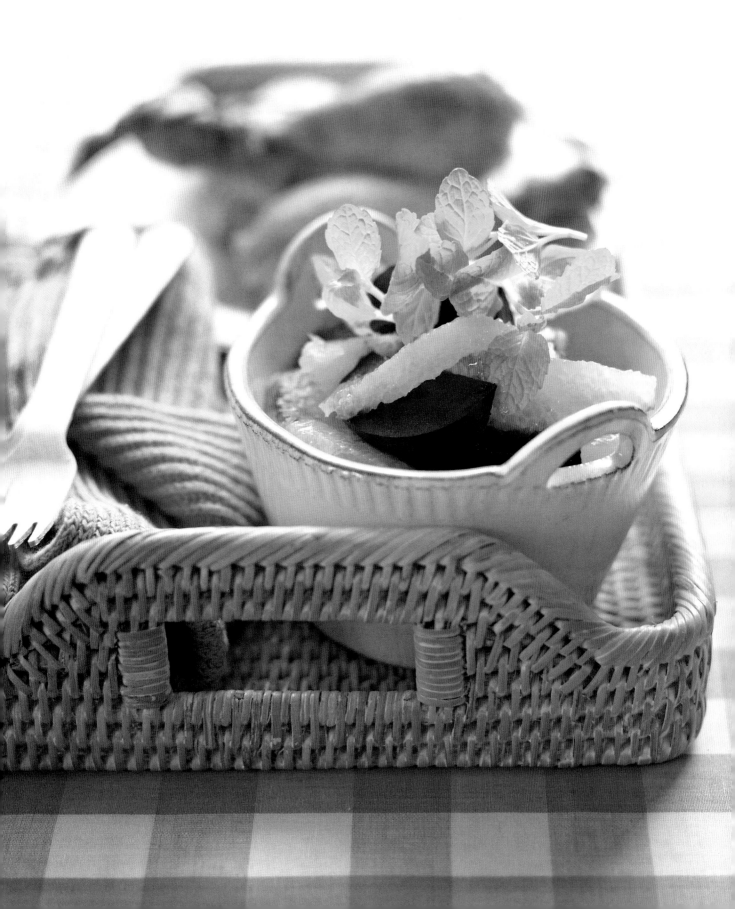

Cold roast beef with horseradish yoghurt

This is wonderful for a picnic, but remember to pack the salad dressing separately and dress it when you're ready to serve or you'll have very soggy watercress!

SERVES 8 | PREP 20 minutes | COOK 30 minutes | COOL 1 hour | CAL PER SERVE 312

1.2 kg beef fillet, at room temperature
2 teaspoons olive oil
freshly ground black pepper
olive oil spray

Horseradish yoghurt
1 cup plain low-cal yoghurt
¼ cup horseradish cream
2 tablespoons finely chopped chives

Watercress salad
1 bunch watercress, leaves picked
400 g can chickpeas, drained
    and rinsed
2 Lebanese cucumbers, sliced
250 g cherry tomatoes, halved
1½ tablespoons olive oil
1 tablespoon red-wine vinegar

1. Preheat your oven to 230°C.

2. Rub the beef fillet with the olive oil and season with pepper. Lightly spray a frying pan with more oil and heat on high, then sear the beef on each side until browned. Transfer to a roasting pan fitted with a wire rack, and roast for 25 minutes for rare (or longer to your desired doneness). Remove from the oven, cover loosely with foil and allow to cool to room temperature before slicing thinly.

3. To make the horseradish yoghurt, combine all the ingredients in a medium bowl and refrigerate until ready to serve.

4. For the salad, combine the watercress, chickpeas, cucumber and tomatoes in a large salad bowl. Drizzle with the olive oil and vinegar, and toss to coat.

5. Serve the roast beef slices with the salad and a dollop of horseradish yoghurt.

TIPS: It's better not to refrigerate the cooked beef if possible, as its flavour will fade in the cold.

• This horseradish yoghurt is quite peppery – if you prefer things milder, go for only 2 tablespoons of horseradish cream.

Za'atar lamb cutlets with tomato and bean salad

The perfect dish for a summer barbecue. I can't go past the heavenly aroma of za'atar.

SERVES 6 | **PREP** 20 minutes | **COOK** 10 minutes | **CAL PER SERVE** 294

18 small frenched lamb cutlets, trimmed of fat
2 tablespoons za'atar

Tomato and bean salad
1 bunch asparagus, trimmed and cut into chunks
150 g green beans
150 g yellow beans
150 g snowpeas, trimmed
250 g yellow and red cherry tomatoes, halved
2 tablespoons shredded mint
freshly ground black pepper

Dressing
1½ tablespoons extra virgin olive oil
1 tablespoon lemon juice

1. Sprinkle the lamb with the za'atar.

2. Bring a large saucepan of water to the boil and cook the asparagus and beans for 2 minutes. Add the snowpeas, cook for another minute, then drain and cool the vegetables in ice-water. Drain again and place in a large salad bowl with the tomatoes and mint.

3. Preheat your barbecue grill or flat plate on high, then cook the lamb cutlets for 1–2 minutes each side for rare (or to the desired doneness). Transfer to a platter and stand, loosely covered with foil, for 5 minutes.

4. To make the dressing, combine the olive oil and lemon juice. Drizzle the dressing over the salad, season with freshly ground black pepper and toss to coat, before serving with the lamb cutlets.

TIP: If you're making this for a barbecue in the park, bring olive oil spray and a sheet of foil to line the barbecue. That way your lamb won't pick up the flavour of whatever was cooked previously on the hotplate (could have been fish!) and you don't have to clean the barbecue afterward.

Asian coleslaw salad

Crunchy, zesty, nutty – this huge coleslaw is just delicious. You can eat it as is, or try serving it with the Chicken meatloaf on page 63 (divided among 8 people, it has 356 cal per serve).

SERVES 4 | **PREP** 15 minutes | **CAL PER SERVE** 285

800 g wombok (chinese cabbage), shredded
2 red capsicums, shredded
2 large carrots, shredded
80 g snowpea sprouts
2 bunches coriander, leaves picked
½ cup mint leaves
½ cup roasted peanuts, coarsely chopped

Dressing
½ cup lime juice
2 tablespoons brown sugar
2 tablespoons fish sauce
1 tablespoon peanut oil
2 teaspoons sesame oil
2 cloves garlic, crushed

1. Combine the wombok, capsicum, carrot, sprouts and herbs in a very large bowl.

2. To make the dressing, combine the juice, sugar, fish sauce, oils and garlic in a small bowl, and stir until the sugar dissolves. Pour the mixture over the salad and toss to coat.

3. Serve sprinkled with peanuts.

TIP: This makes a great picnic dish. You can either dress the salad at home (it will wilt slightly) or at the picnic for maximum crunch, but make sure you only add the peanuts when you're ready to serve or they'll go soggy.

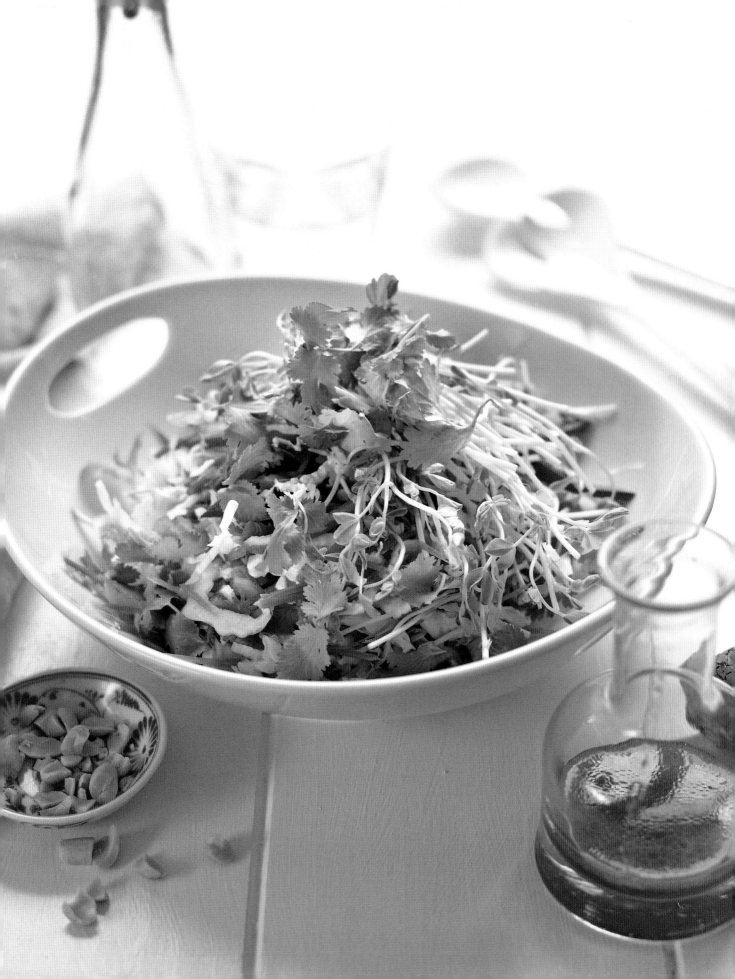

Asparagus, rocket and ricotta frittata

This is wonderful for a barbecue or picnic – just make sure you let it cool before you wrap it in foil or plastic film or it'll go soggy.

SERVES 4 | **PREP** 15 minutes | **COOK** 25 minutes | **CAL PER SERVE** 273

olive oil spray
1 bunch asparagus, trimmed
   and cut into 4 cm pieces
8 eggs
½ cup finely grated parmesan

1 cup low-cal ricotta, crumbled
freshly ground black pepper
40 g rocket, coarsely chopped
2 tablespoons chopped basil

1. Preheat your oven to 180°C. Lightly oil and line a 16 cm × 26 cm slice pan with baking paper.

2. Bring a small saucepan of salted water to the boil and cook the asparagus for 1–2 minutes or until just tender and bright green. Drain and cool in ice-water, then drain again.

3. In a large bowl, whisk the eggs, parmesan and two-thirds of the ricotta until smooth. Season with pepper, then stir in the rocket, basil and asparagus.

4. Pour the mixture into your prepared pan, making sure that the asparagus and rocket are evenly distributed. Dot with spoonfuls of the remaining ricotta and bake for 20 minutes or until golden and set.

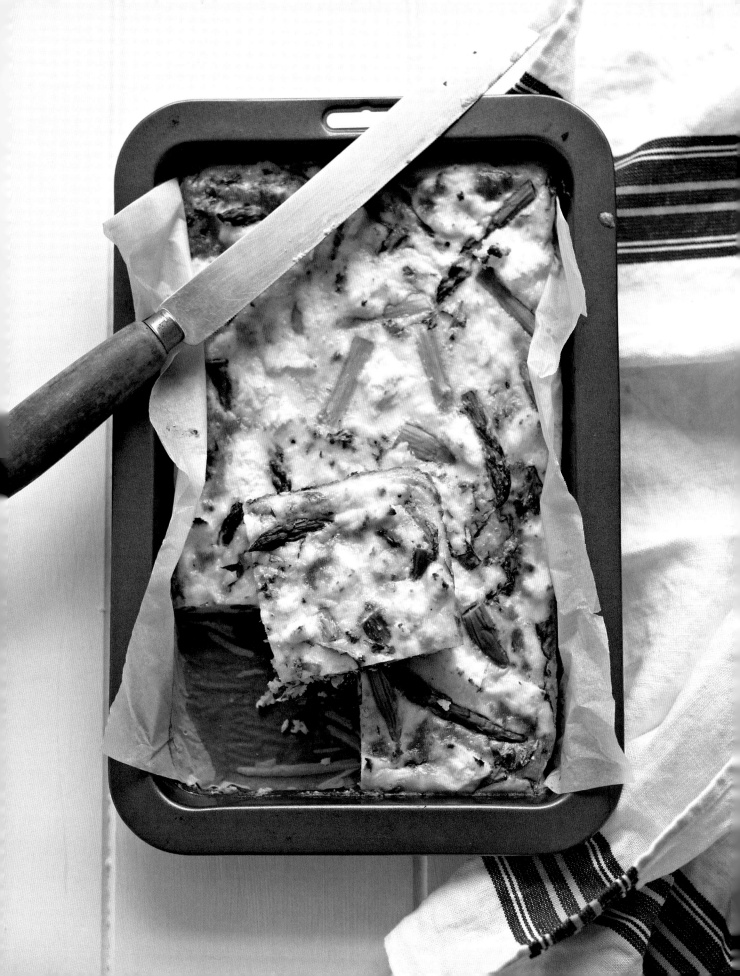

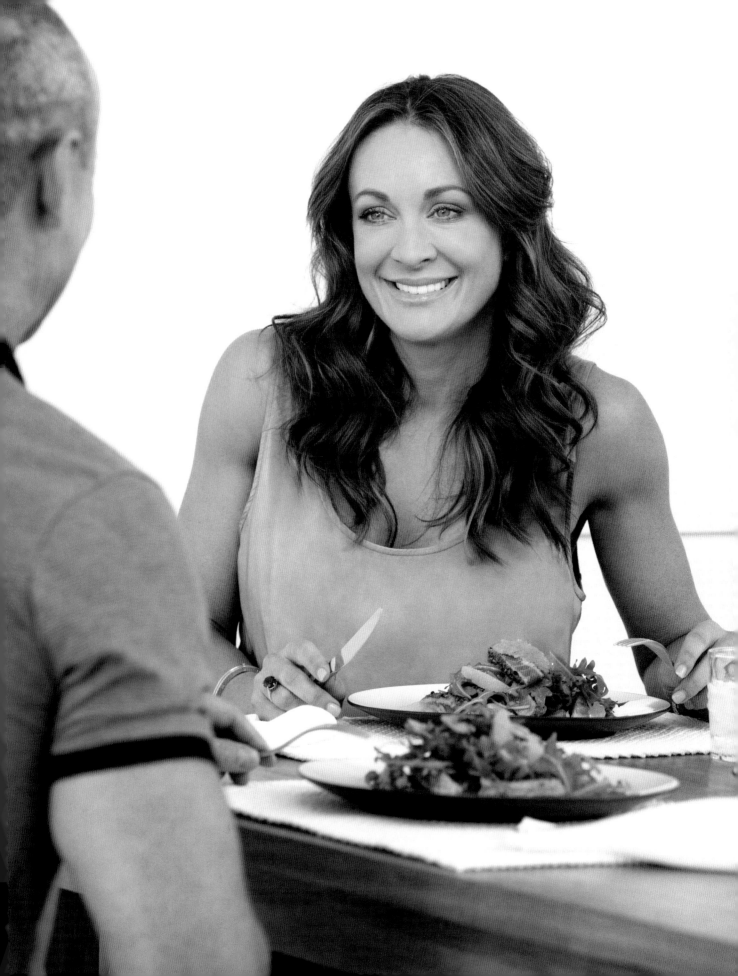

dinner

Prawn, mango and avocado salad

Prawns and mango make this salad an everyday luxury. It's also brilliant to serve in smaller portions as a starter at a dinner party.

SERVES 2 | **PREP** 15 minutes | **CAL PER SERVE** 321

½ small iceberg lettuce, thickly sliced
1 medium avocado, sliced
1 small mango, sliced
14 cooked king prawns, peeled and
  deveined, tails intact
2 tablespoons snipped chives

Dressing
1 tablespoon lemon juice
2 teaspoons extra virgin olive oil
Tabasco, to taste
freshly ground black pepper

1. To make the dressing, combine the lemon juice, olive oil and Tabasco in a small bowl. Season with pepper.

2. Arrange the lettuce, avocado, mango and prawns on two plates and drizzle with the dressing. Sprinkle with chives to serve.

TIP: If you want to, you could buy green king prawns and cook them yourself. Just bring a medium saucepan of salted water to the boil, add the prawns and reduce the heat to a gentle simmer. Cook for about 3 minutes or until the prawns are pink and opaque, then drain and cool before peeling. You can also reserve the cooking liquid, reduce it to concentrate its flavour and use it in a fish soup – just make sure to freeze it once it's cooled if you're not using it straight away.

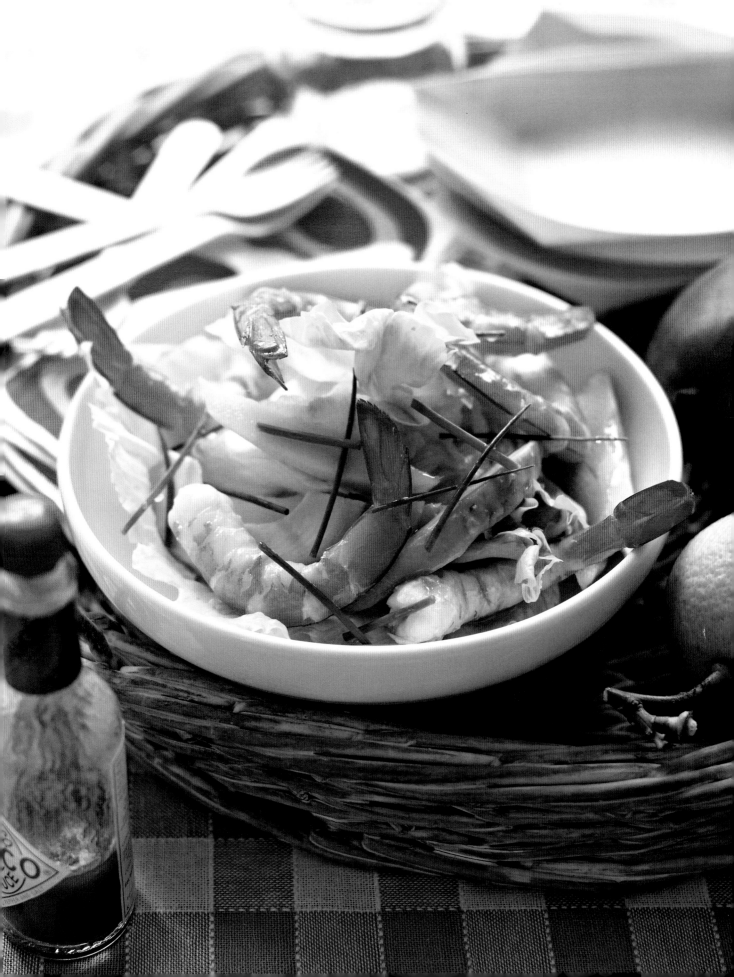

Endive, walnut, blue cheese and apple salad

This endive salad reminds me of when I lived in France. You don't have to give up blue-cheese dressing to be healthy!

SERVES 2 | **PREP** 15 minutes | **CAL PER SERVE** 310

250 g endive, cored
  and roughly chopped
1 red apple, peel on, cored
  and thinly sliced
⅓ cup coarsely chopped walnuts
freshly ground black pepper

Dressing
¼ cup buttermilk
2 teaspoons Dijon mustard
½ teaspoon red-wine vinegar
50 g sharp blue cheese, crumbled
2 tablespoons chopped chives

1. To make the dressing, combine the buttermilk, mustard, vinegar and half of the blue cheese in a small bowl and mix with a fork until smooth. Stir in half of the chives.

2. Arrange the endive, apple, walnuts and the remaining blue cheese on a large platter, drizzle with the dressing and sprinkle over the remaining chives. Season with pepper and serve immediately.

TIPS: To give this salad more volume, just separate the endive leaves and add them whole.

• Endives are deliciously peppery, and the greener their leaves, the stronger the flavour. Choose greener or paler endives according to your taste.

Warm roasted tomato salad

For a bigger meal, serve this salad for two with a 220 g grilled white fish fillet (360 cal per serve) or a 175 g grilled chicken breast (366 cal per serve).

SERVES 2 | PREP 15 minutes | COOK 45 minutes | CAL PER SERVE 227

6 roma tomatoes
freshly ground black pepper
2 teaspoons olive oil
1 long red chilli, finely chopped
1 clove garlic, thinly sliced

400 g can chickpeas,
  drained and rinsed
¼ teaspoon ground cumin
¼ teaspoon ground coriander
150 g baby spinach leaves
1 tablespoon lemon juice

1. Preheat your oven to 180°C.

2. Prick the tomatoes all over, then halve them lengthwise and place them on a wire rack. Season with pepper and roast in the oven for 45 minutes.

3. Meanwhile, heat the olive oil in a large frying pan on medium and cook the chilli and garlic for 1 minute. Add the chickpeas and spices and cook until fragrant, then stir in the spinach and lemon juice and cook until wilted. Season with pepper to taste.

4. Toss the tomatoes through the chickpea and spinach mixture to serve.

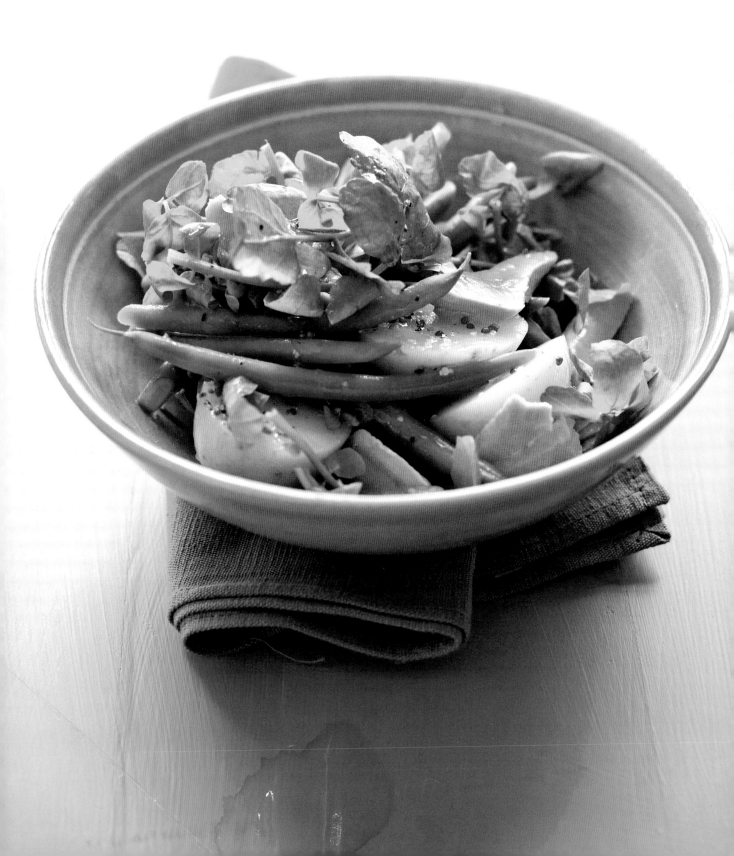

Poached ocean trout salad

Poaching is my all-time favourite way of preparing fish and chicken –
no more dry, tasteless flesh! And it's definitely worth chasing up the
watercress at your local market in spring, early summer and autumn
if you can't find it at the supermarket: it adds a lovely peppery flavour.

SERVES 2 | **PREP** 15 minutes | **COOK** 25 minutes | **CAL PER SERVE** 300

150 g new potatoes, halved
2 tablespoons white-wine vinegar
2 teaspoons extra virgin olive oil
2 teaspoons wholegrain mustard
freshly ground black pepper

4 sprigs dill
250 g ocean trout, skin on
100 g green beans, trimmed
1 bunch watercress, leaves washed
  and picked

1. Put the potatoes in a medium saucepan, cover them with water and bring to the boil. Boil for 12 minutes or until tender when pricked with a fork, then drain and slice. Place in a large bowl and drizzle with 2 teaspoons of the vinegar while still warm.

2. Meanwhile, combine the olive oil, mustard and 2 teaspoons of vinegar in a small bowl. Season with pepper.

3. Half-fill a small shallow saucepan with water and add the remaining tablespoon of vinegar and the dill. Bring to a gentle simmer, reduce the heat to low and simmer for 5 minutes. Lower the trout gently into the poaching liquid and return it to a simmer. Cook for 2–3 minutes until the fish is firm to touch and the flesh is opaque, then remove it from the pan with a slotted spoon. Discard the poaching liquid. Discard the skin and flake the fish when it's cool enough to handle.

4. While the fish is cooking, bring a small saucepan of salted water to the boil and add the green beans. Boil for 2 minutes until just tender and bright green, drain and cool in ice-water, then drain again.

5. Add the beans, watercress and ocean trout to the potatoes. Drizzle with the dressing and gently toss to coat.

Kangaroo, beetroot and feta salad

My favourite meat needs no introduction! When cooked correctly,
it's tender and surprisingly delicate in flavour.

SERVES 2 | **PREP** 15 minutes | **COOK** 5 minutes | **CAL PER SERVE** 272

100 g mesclun salad mix, washed
440 g can baby beetroot,
   drained and halved
50 g feta, crumbled

2 teaspoons olive oil
200 g kangaroo fillet, trimmed
freshly ground black pepper
1 tablespoon white-wine vinegar

1. Combine the mesclun, beetroot and feta
   in a large bowl.

2. Heat the olive oil in a large frying pan
   on high. Season the kangaroo with pepper,
   and cook it for 1–2 minutes on each side
   until well browned but still rare. Remove
   from the pan and stand for 2 minutes
   before slicing.

3. Add the kangaroo and vinegar to the
   bowl of salad and toss to coat.

TIPS: If you prefer to keep the feta white,
sprinkle it over the salad at the end rather
than mixing it with the beetroot and
mesclun.

• Make sure the pan is really hot before
you cook the kangaroo – it needs to be
cooked rare or medium to be tender.
Also, while kangaroo meat doesn't have
any fat, make sure to trim off any sinew,
as it can be chewy.

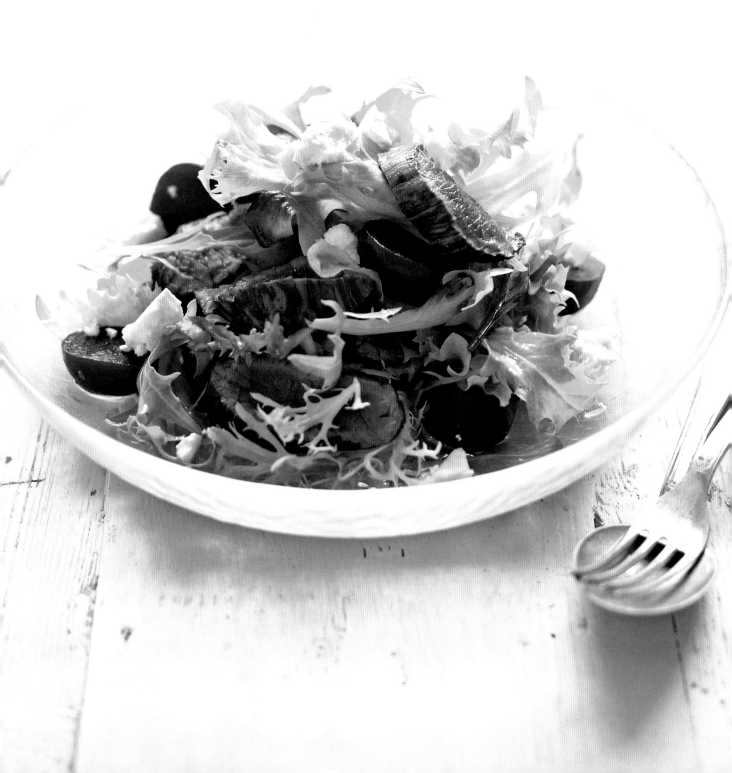

Salmon stir-fry with gai lan and water chestnuts

Stir-fries are an absolute basic in our house. You might not think of using salmon in one, but in fact the high heat and quick cooking result in a nicely seared crust and a beautiful rare interior. Luscious!

SERVES 2 | **PREP** 10 minutes | **COOK** 10 minutes | **CAL PER SERVE** 291

2 teaspoons peanut oil
3 cloves garlic, sliced
1 bunch asparagus,
    cut into 4 cm chunks
227 g can water chestnuts,
    drained and rinsed

1 bunch gai lan, washed, stems
    coarsely chopped and leaves torn
250 g salmon fillet, skin off, deboned
    and cut into 3 cm cubes
1½ tablespoons lemon juice
3 teaspoons low-salt soy sauce

1. Heat half the oil in a wok or medium frying pan on medium, and stir-fry the garlic for 3 minutes or until golden. Remove from the wok with a slotted spoon.

2. Increase the heat to high. Stir-fry the asparagus, water chestnuts and gai lan stems for 4–5 minutes or until just tender, then remove them from the wok.

3. Heat the remaining oil and stir-fry the salmon cubes until browned but still pink inside. Add the lemon juice and stir-fry for a further 30 seconds, or until the juice has almost evaporated. Remove from the wok.

4. Stir-fry the gai lan leaves until they start to wilt, then return all the ingredients to the wok with the soy sauce and stir-fry until coated. Serve immediately.

TIP: Make sure you don't cut the salmon cubes too small, or they'll overcook and be dry.

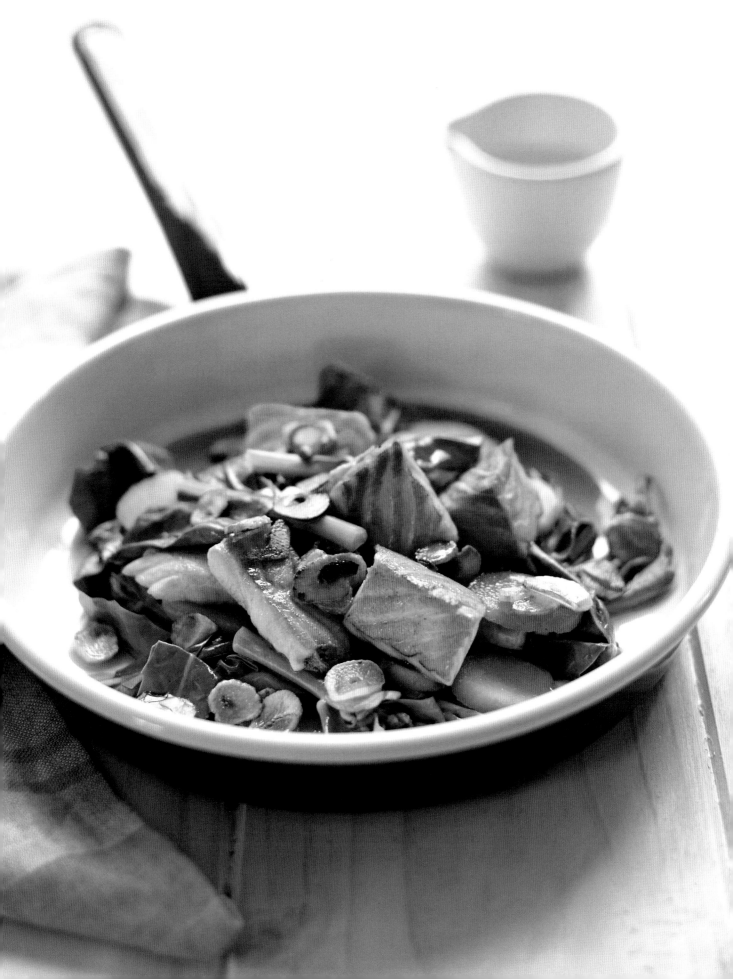

Thai chilli prawn stir-fry

You can remove the prawns' heads if they freak you out,
but many people consider them the best part . . . up to you!

SERVES 2 | **PREP** 20 minutes | **COOK** 10 minutes | **CAL PER SERVE** 246

2 teaspoons peanut oil
1 bunch broccolini, trimmed
   and cut into chunks
1 bunch asparagus, trimmed
   and cut into chunks
1 green capsicum, sliced
500 g green prawns, peeled and
   deveined, tails and heads intact

25 g ginger, peeled and
   thinly sliced
1 small red chilli, sliced
1 cup torn Thai basil leaves
3 teaspoons fish sauce
½ teaspoon brown sugar
2 teaspoons lime juice

1. Heat half the oil in a wok on medium–high, and stir-fry the broccolini, asparagus and capsicum for 5 minutes until just tender. Remove them from the wok.

2. Heat the remaining oil in the wok on high. Stir-fry the prawns and ginger for 3 minutes, until the prawns are pink and opaque. Add the chilli and half of the basil, and stir-fry for another minute. Tip the vegetables back into the wok, add the fish sauce, sugar and lime juice, and toss to coat.

3. Transfer the stir-fry to a serving bowl and scatter with the remaining basil.

Leek and tarragon mussels

This is my take on the French and Belgian classic *moules marinière*
(sailor's mussels). Just skip the traditional accompaniment of
French fries and mayo!

SERVES 2 | **PREP** 20 minutes | **COOK** 10 minutes | **CAL PER SERVE** 355

1 kg mussels
1 teaspoon olive oil
1 leek, cut into matchsticks
1 clove garlic, crushed

⅓ cup dry white wine
¼ cup torn tarragon leaves
2 slices wholemeal bread

1. Scrub the mussels under cold water and remove the beards (the stringy stuff trailing from the shell). Discard any that are cracked or that don't shut when you tap them.

2. Heat the olive oil in a large saucepan on medium and cook the leek and garlic for 2 minutes until they start to soften. Increase the heat to high, then add the mussels, the wine and half of the tarragon leaves. Cover and cook for 4 minutes or until the mussels open, stirring halfway through.

3. Meanwhile, put the bread on to toast.

4. Serve the mussels immediately in shallow bowls, with their cooking liquid. Sprinkle them with the remaining tarragon and serve the toast on the side.

TIPS: If you don't want to remove the mussel beards yourself, ready-scrubbed bags of mussels are usually available at fishmongers.

• According to the Australian Mussel Industry Association, it's a myth that you need to discard mussels that don't open during cooking – they're perfectly safe. You *do*, however, need to get rid of any that don't close when tapped before you cook them.

Thai chicken larb

I love the clean, zingy flavours in this dish. It's great to put
in a lunch box as well.

SERVES 2 | **PREP** 20 minutes | **COOK** 5 minutes | **CAL PER SERVE** 301

juice of half a lime
3 teaspoons fish sauce
½ teaspoon brown sugar
2 teaspoons peanut oil
1 lemongrass stalk, pale part only,
  finely chopped
1 birdseye chilli, finely chopped
1 clove garlic, crushed
300 g lean chicken mince

1 red shallot, thinly sliced
⅓ cup coriander leaves
⅓ cup mint leaves
½ Lebanese cucumber, shaved into
  ribbons with a vegetable peeler
½ iceberg lettuce, leaves separated
  and trimmed into cups
lime wedges, to serve

1. Combine the lime juice, fish sauce
   and sugar in a bowl and set aside.

2. Heat the oil in a wok on medium and
   stir-fry the lemongrass, chilli and garlic
   for 1 minute until fragrant. Remove from
   the wok.

3. Stir-fry the chicken for 4 minutes until
   brown, stirring to break up any lumps.
   Return the lemongrass mixture to the
   wok, add the lime juice mixture, shallot
   and herbs, and toss to combine.

4. Serve the larb with the cucumber in the
   lettuce cups, with lime wedges on the side.

TIP: This is a spicy salad, so you may
want to start with half a chilli – you can
always add the rest after you've tasted
the mixture.

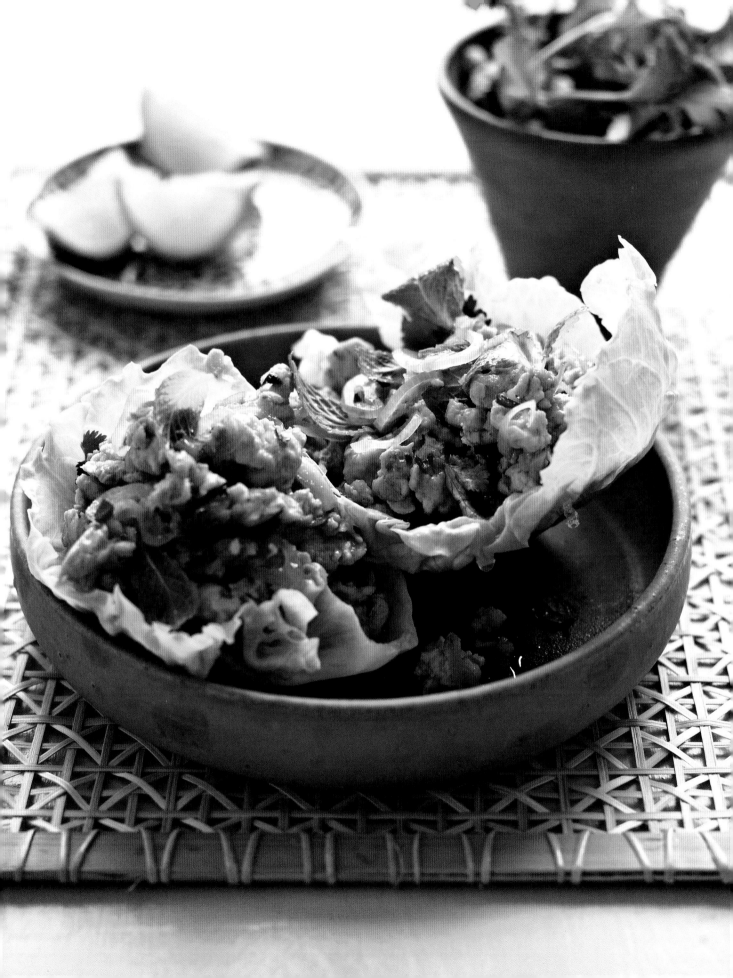

Miso chicken skewers with steamed Asian veggies

This miso marinade is magic. Don't stop at chicken; make up a big batch and use it on everything – steak, pork, oily fish. It's a winner.

SERVES 2 | **PREP** 20 minutes | **COOK** 5 minutes | **CAL PER SERVE** 289

300 g chicken thigh fillet,
   trimmed of fat, cut into strips
cooking oil spray
1 bunch broccolini, trimmed
1 bunch asparagus, trimmed
1 bunch gai lan, trimmed
   and leaves separated
2 spring onions, cut into matchsticks

Miso marinade
1 tablespoon red miso
1 tablespoon lime juice
2 teaspoons finely grated ginger
1 teaspoon low-salt soy sauce
1 teaspoon peanut oil

1. To make the miso marinade, combine all the ingredients with 1 tablespoon of water in a large bowl. Reserve 1½ tablespoons. Place the chicken in the marinade and toss to coat, then thread it onto small skewers. Put a saucepan of water on to boil.

2. Lightly spray a char-grill pan with oil and heat on medium–high. Cook the chicken for 5 minutes, turning regularly until it starts to caramelise and is just cooked through.

3. Meanwhile, steam the broccolini over the saucepan of boiling water for 2 minutes. Add the asparagus and gai lan, and steam for another 2 minutes until the asparagus is just tender and the leaves are wilted.

4. To serve, drizzle the reserved marinade over the steamed vegetables, top with spring onion, and place the chicken skewers on the side.

Pepper kangaroo stir-fry

Kangaroo is lean, free-range, killed humanely and tastes terrific. It really is a super-food, and is shown to its best advantage in this quick stir-fry.

SERVES 2 | PREP 15 minutes | COOK 10 minutes | CAL PER SERVE 310

2 teaspoons peanut oil
2 brown onions, cut into wedges
1 large red capsicum, cut into strips
300 g green beans, trimmed
300 g kangaroo fillet, trimmed
   and thinly sliced

1 teaspoon freshly ground
   black pepper
2 teaspoons low-salt soy sauce
malt vinegar, to serve (optional)

1. Heat half the oil in a wok on high, then stir-fry the onion and capsicum for 3–4 minutes until just tender. Remove them from the wok.

2. Heat the remaining oil and stir-fry the beans for 5 minutes until just tender. Remove from the wok.

3. Season the kangaroo with the pepper and stir-fry for 30 seconds, then return the vegetables to the wok, add the soy sauce, and toss to coat.

4. Serve drizzled with a little malt vinegar if you like.

TIP: Make sure the wok is really hot for the kangaroo and only stir-fry it until just seared, or you'll overcook it and make it tough.

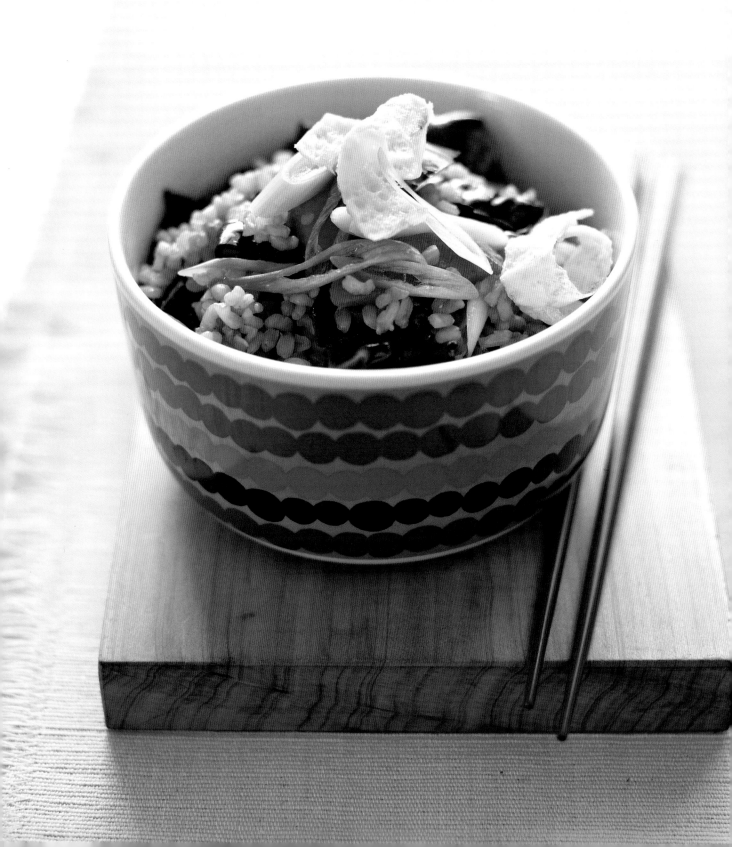

'Rainbow' fried brown rice

You don't have to give up your favourite dishes to be healthy – tweak a fried-rice recipe with a few extra veggies and go easy on the oil, and you can eat it as often as you like.

SERVES 2 | **PREP** 15 minutes | **COOK** 35 minutes | **CAL PER SERVE** 316

½ cup medium-grain brown rice
2 teaspoons peanut oil
1 egg, lightly beaten
1 carrot, halved lengthwise
   and sliced on the diagonal
1 green capsicum, chopped
   into chunks

100 g red cabbage, coarsely shredded
1 clove garlic, crushed
2 spring onions, sliced on the diagonal
3 teaspoons low-salt soy sauce
½ long red chilli, sliced
   on the diagonal

1. Cook the rice in a small saucepan of boiling water for 25 minutes or until tender, then drain and rinse under cold water. Drain well.

2. Heat a non-stick wok on medium–high. Add the oil, swirl it and tip it out into a bowl. Add the egg and swirl it around the wok to make a very thin omelette: cook for 30 seconds or until set. Slide the omelette onto a clean board, roll it tightly and slice into thin strips.

3. Return the oil to the wok and stir-fry the carrot and capsicum for 4 minutes until just tender. Add the cabbage and stir-fry for another 2 minutes, then add the garlic and half the spring onion and stir-fry until fragrant. Add the rice and soy sauce and stir-fry until heated through.

4. Serve garnished with the omelette strips, chilli slices and the remaining spring onion.

TIP: If you cook the rice ahead of time, this becomes a very quick stir-fry!

Beef and oyster sauce stir-fry

Quick, healthy and very more-ish – watch your portion sizes!

SERVES 2 | **PREP** 15 minutes | **COOK** 10 minutes | **CAL PER SERVE** 343

2 teaspoons peanut oil
1 bunch broccolini,
   cut into 4 cm chunks
1 red onion, cut into wedges
125 g baby sweet corn, halved
   lengthwise on the diagonal
175 g rump steak, fat trimmed, sliced

250 g mixed mushrooms
   (brown, oyster, etc.), chopped
2 cloves garlic, crushed
3 cm piece ginger, peeled
   and shredded
1½ tablespoons oyster sauce

1. Heat half the oil in a wok on high and stir-fry the broccolini, onion and corn for 5 minutes or until just tender. Remove from the wok.

2. Heat the remaining oil in the wok, add the beef and stir-fry until just browned. Remove from the wok.

3. Stir-fry the mushrooms, garlic and ginger for 3–4 minutes or until they're browned and the moisture has evaporated. Return the vegetables and beef to the wok, add the oyster sauce and stir-fry until well coated.

TIPS: You can halve or quarter the mushrooms, depending on the size.

• It's important to just sear the beef, or it will overcook and be tough.

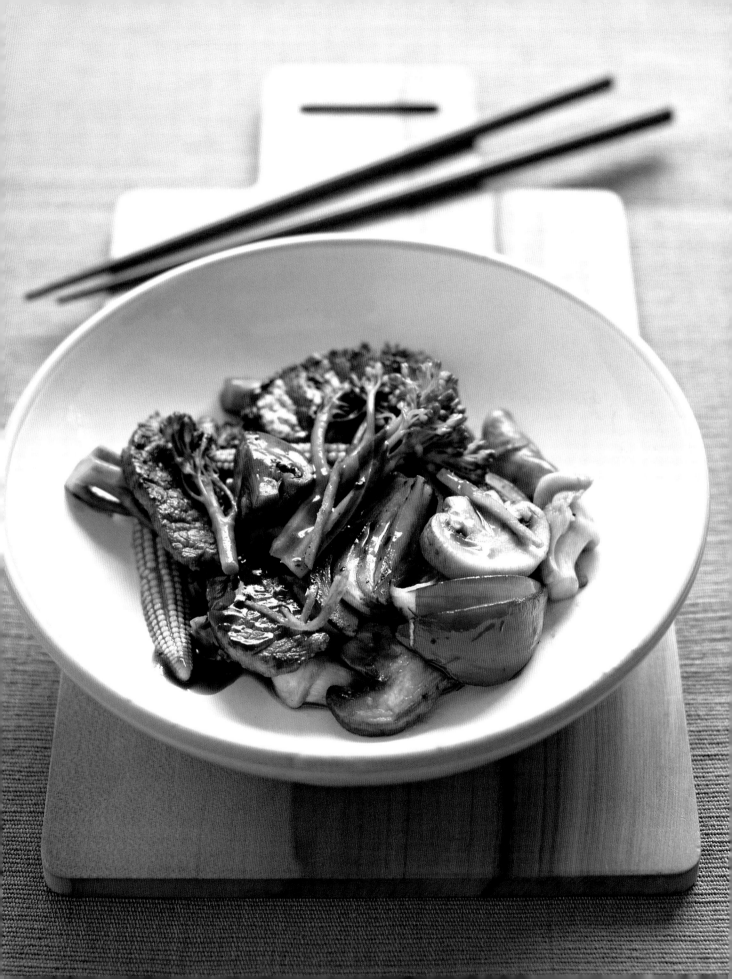

Hoisin chicken, pumpkin and celery stir-fry

Pumpkin and celery actually cook beautifully in a wok, as long as you slice them thinly. The fast cooking retains maximum nutrients.

SERVES 2 | **PREP** 15 minutes | **COOK** 15 minutes | **CAL PER SERVE** 331

2 teaspoons peanut oil
300 g pumpkin, peeled, seeded and thinly sliced into wedges
2 stalks celery, trimmed and sliced on the diagonal
6 spring onions, trimmed and cut into large pieces
250 g chicken breast, skin off, thinly sliced
1 tablespoon hoisin sauce
1 tablespoon chopped coriander

1. Heat half the oil in a non-stick wok on medium–high and stir-fry the pumpkin for 5 minutes until just tender. Remove from the wok. Stir-fry the celery and spring onion for 2–3 minutes until just tender, then remove them from the wok.

2. Heat the remaining oil in the wok and stir-fry the chicken for 3 minutes until just cooked through. Return the vegetables to the wok with the hoisin sauce, and toss to coat and warm through.

3. Serve sprinkled with the coriander.

Kate from Brisbane, 32

Starting weight: 108.9 kg

At the time of writing: 86.5 kg

I had all the wrong habits, born out of pure laziness and my excuse of being 'too busy'. I often had no breakfast, ate a late lunch and then a late dinner. Because I hadn't fed myself well during the day, my dinners would usually be big portions and high in calories, and I'd often pick at high-calorie food right through to bedtime. I have a night job as a singer, so I'd also often miss dinner but eat lots of the fried finger food on offer at work.

It became a habit NOT to cook. We'd have take-out probably three or four nights a week, always eating out of a bowl, on the couch. I feel like that's a lifestyle many of us have fallen into – eating on the couch, out of a bowl, no knife, just a fork.

I enjoy cooking now. I enjoy the fact that I'm the one getting my health back on track. Yes, I spend more time in the kitchen, but it's organised and highly time-efficient. Michelle's recipes are so easy, I find it exciting to make a new dish, and I don't feel like I'm being deprived. I make time to cook up food for the freezer, so I'm never caught out when I come home late. I always have fruit in my bag and I think ahead so I don't end up succumbing to temptation if there are no healthy choices around.

And now, when I say no to certain foods I actually mean it, whereas in the past I might have said no to biscuits or cake but deep down still really wanted them. I can also now appreciate a beautiful meal out, sharing a dish: not ordering every-thing off the menu and eating like it's the Last Supper! That's quite a powerful thing to acknowledge. I am a different woman, and life is great!

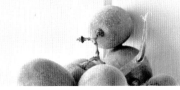

Portuguese chicken with grilled capsicum salad

This is a really special dish for a weekend lunch or dinner party.

SERVES 6 | **PREP** 30 minutes | **MARINATE** 30 minutes | **COOK** 50 minutes | **CAL PER SERVE** 326

3 long red chillies, chopped
4 cloves garlic, chopped
2 teaspoons extra virgin olive oil
zest and juice of 1 lemon
2 teaspoons dried oregano
1.6 kg whole chicken, skin removed

Grilled capsicum salad
1 red capsicum
1 green capsicum
400 g ripe tomatoes, sliced
½ brown onion, thinly sliced into rings
1 tablespoon extra virgin olive oil
1 tablespoon white-wine vinegar
freshly ground black pepper

1. Preheat your barbecue on medium. For this recipe, you'll need a barbecue with a lid for roasting the chicken; alternatively, you can use a hot grill placed so that the chicken is about 10–15 cm from the element.

2. Combine the chilli, garlic, olive oil and lemon zest and juice in a small food processor and process until smooth. Transfer to a shallow dish and stir in the dried oregano. (You'll be using this mixture to marinate your chicken.) Reserve 1 tablespoon of the marinade in a separate dish.

3. Using a sharp knife, cut along both sides of the chicken's breastbone, as close as you can to the bone to avoid any waste. Then with sharp kitchen scissors, cut away the breastbone. Place the chicken breast-side up on a clean board and press down to flatten. Using a knife, cut a few slits through the thicker parts of the breast and leg, then place the chicken on a plate and rub with the marinade. Stand for 30 minutes.

4. Meanwhile, make the salad. Put the whole capsicums under a preheated grill for 10 minutes, turning regularly as the skin blackens. While still hot, place them in a plastic bag, tie a knot to close it and stand for 10 minutes to sweat and cool slightly. Remove them from the bag, discard the skin, seeds and membrane and thickly slice the capsicum flesh.

5. Arrange the capsicum and tomato slices on a large plate and top with the onion. Drizzle with oil and vinegar, then grind over some pepper.

6. Grill the chicken on the barbecue breast-side down for about 5 minutes. Then turn it breast-side up and cook with the barbecue lid down for 30–35 minutes or until just cooked through. Brush with the reserved marinade, turn, and barbecue breast-side down again for 30 seconds. Remove from the barbecue, cover loosely with foil and stand for 10 minutes. Carve the chicken and serve with the grilled capsicum salad.

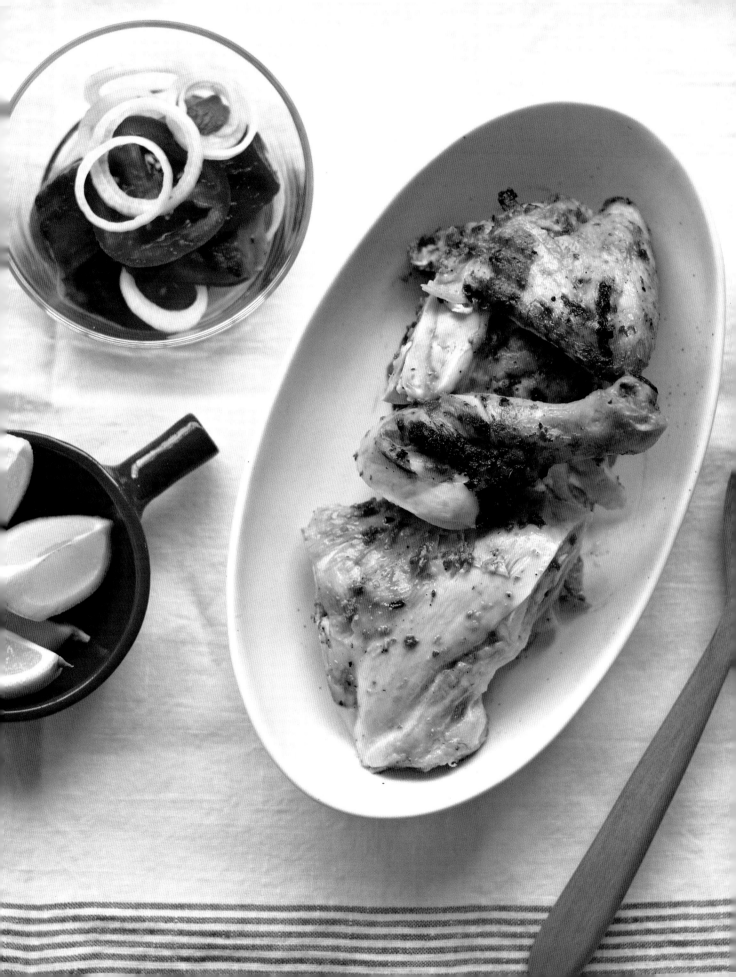

Char-grilled chicken with green papaya salad

If you haven't tried green papaya before, don't hesitate. It has a crisp, chewy texture and mild taste that's superb for carrying stronger flavours. Green papaya salad is a Thai hawker staple.

SERVES 2 | **PREP** 15 minutes | **COOK** 10 minutes | **CAL PER SERVE** 339

olive oil spray
200 g chicken breast, skin off
freshly ground black pepper
2 tablespoons chopped roasted
    peanuts

Green papaya salad
450 g green papaya, peeled, seeded
    and shredded
200 g cherry tomatoes, halved

100 g bean sprouts, trimmed
2 spring onions, trimmed and thinly
    sliced on the diagonal
1 cup torn Thai basil leaves

Dressing
2 tablespoons lime juice
1 tablespoon fish sauce
2 teaspoons low-salt soy sauce
2 teaspoons brown sugar

1. To make the salad, place the papaya, tomatoes, sprouts, spring onion and basil in a salad bowl. Combine the dressing ingredients in a small bowl and stir until the sugar dissolves.

2. Lightly spray a char-grill with olive oil and heat on medium–high. Season the chicken with freshly ground black pepper, then grill for 8 minutes, turning halfway through, until lightly charred and just cooked through. Thinly slice the chicken.

3. Drizzle the dressing over the salad, gently toss to coat, and divide it between two bowls. Top each salad with chicken and sprinkle with peanuts to serve.

Lemon and oregano chicken skewers with red coleslaw

The coleslaw alone is only 135 cal per serve. Why not make a double batch and wrap the leftovers in two slices of Mountain Bread for your lunch boxes (200 cal per serve)?

SERVES 2 | PREP 30 minutes | COOK 10 minutes | CAL PER SERVE 347

250 g chicken breast, skin off,
   cut into 2 cm cubes
2 tablespoons coarsely
   chopped oregano
2 teaspoons lemon zest
1 tablespoon lemon juice
2 teaspoons olive oil
freshly ground black pepper

Red coleslaw
200 g red cabbage, finely shredded
½ green capsicum, shredded
2 spring onions, shredded

Dressing
2 tablespoons wholegrain mustard
1 tablespoon extra virgin olive oil
1 tablespoon red-wine vinegar

1. Combine the chicken, oregano, zest, juice and olive oil in a medium bowl. Season with pepper, toss to coat, then let stand for 10 minutes. Thread the chicken onto skewers.

2. Preheat your barbecue grill on medium and cook the chicken for 10 minutes, turning regularly, until it's lightly charred and just cooked.

3. Meanwhile, combine the dressing ingredients in a small bowl. Combine the coleslaw ingredients in a large bowl, drizzle with the dressing and toss to coat.

4. Serve the chicken skewers with a side of coleslaw.

TIP: If you're using bamboo skewers, make sure you soak them in cold water for 15 minutes so they don't scorch when you cook the chicken.

Moroccan vegetable and couscous salad

This quick couscous makes a great addition to your lunch box during the week – try making a double batch and refrigerating the leftovers in two airtight containers. It's delicious at room temperature, or heat it up in the microwave.

SERVES 2 | PREP 15 minutes | COOK 10 minutes | CAL PER SERVE 299

olive oil spray
1 red capsicum, cut into large wedges
1 red onion, cut into large wedges
1 large zucchini, thickly sliced
   on the diagonal
1½ tablespoons Moroccan seasoning

3 roma tomatoes, halved
½ cup couscous
2 tablespoons finely chopped mint
2 tablespoons finely chopped
   flat-leaf parsley
½ cup plain low-cal yoghurt

1. Lightly spray your barbecue's flat plate with olive oil and preheat on medium–high.

2. Place the capsicum, onion and zucchini in a bowl with the seasoning and toss to coat. Transfer to the barbecue and cook for 8 minutes or until lightly charred and tender. Towards the end of the cooking time, add the tomatoes separately to the barbecue and cook for 2 minutes each side or until lightly charred.

3. Meanwhile, combine the couscous with half a cup of boiling water in a medium bowl, and stir until most of the water has been absorbed. Cover and stand for 2 minutes, then fluff the couscous up with a fork and stand again, covered, for another 2 minutes. Fluff it up once more and stir through the herbs, capsicum, onion and zucchini.

4. Serve the couscous with the tomatoes and a dollop of yoghurt.

TIP: If you'd like to add a little chilli heat, mix some harissa in with the yoghurt to serve.

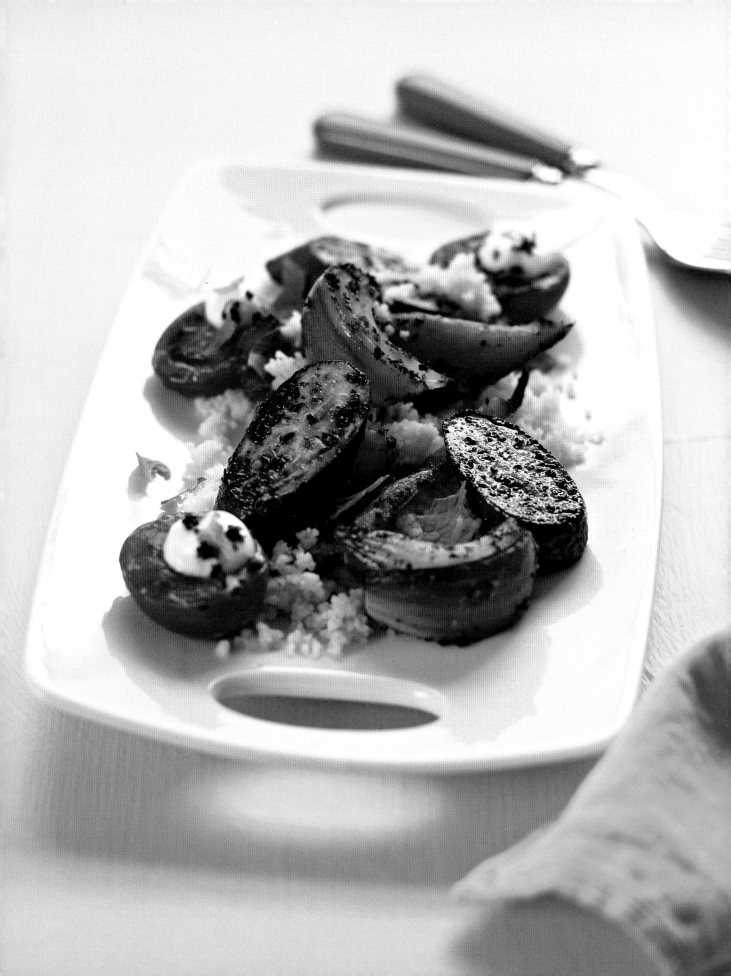

Barbecued ocean trout with dill and apple coleslaw

This is such an easy way to barbecue fish – try substituting your favourite type. Salmon works particularly well.

SERVES 6 | **PREP** 30 minutes | **COOK** 20 minutes | **CAL PER SERVE** 339

1.2 kg whole fillet of ocean trout,
    skin on, deboned
freshly ground black pepper
2 tablespoons chopped dill
half a lemon, sliced
olive oil spray

Dill and apple coleslaw
300 g green cabbage, shredded
1 granny smith apple, unpeeled,
    cut into small batons
2 spring onions, thinly sliced
1 cup plain low-cal yoghurt
1 tablespoon Dijon mustard
2 tablespoons chopped dill
freshly ground black pepper

1. Preheat your barbecue flat plate on high.

2. Place the ocean trout skin-side down on a clean board, then halve it lengthwise and season with pepper. Sprinkle half of the dill over one piece of the trout, top with the lemon slices and sprinkle over the remaining dill. Place the second piece of trout on top, skin-side up, tie the layers together with kitchen string and lightly spray with olive oil.

3. Place 2 large pieces of foil on top of each other on a clean board and cover with a large sheet of baking paper. Arrange the fish in the centre, and enclose first in the paper and then in the foil. Cook the wrapped trout on the barbecue for 20 minutes, turning halfway through.

4. Meanwhile, to make the coleslaw, combine all the ingredients in a large bowl and season with pepper.

5. Carefully unwrap the fish from the foil and paper and slice into 6 portions. Place portions on serving plates, then cut and remove the string. Serve the fish with the coleslaw.

TIPS: A 'whole fillet' is a fillet that runs the full length of the fish. Ask your fishmonger for one if there are none on display.

• The coleslaw makes about 4 cups and is 82 cal per cup.

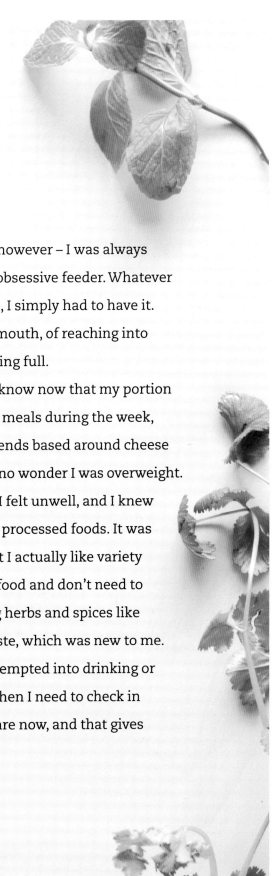

Kerri from Darwin, 39

Starting weight: 64.5 kg

At the time of writing: 55.9 kg

Emotional eating was my thing. Whatever, whenever, however – I was always thinking about what I could eat next. I guess I was an obsessive feeder. Whatever was in the fridge, it wouldn't really matter what it was, I simply had to have it. It wasn't that I was hungry, it was the idea of hand to mouth, of reaching into the fridge. I would usually eat way past the point of being full.

Although to me, my diet seemed healthy enough, I know now that my portion sizes were too big. Add to that a couple of high-calorie meals during the week, some high-calorie snacks, a few junk-food runs, weekends based around cheese and wine, and my emotional-eating habits, and it was no wonder I was overweight.

During the first two weeks on Michelle's meal plan I felt unwell, and I knew I was withdrawing from all the caffeine, sugar, fat and processed foods. It was a wake-up call. Then I started to feel great. I found that I actually like variety in my food. I discovered that I enjoy the taste of fresh food and don't need to cover it with mayonnaise, dressings and sauces. Using herbs and spices like ginger, mint and basil gave food an amazingly fresh taste, which was new to me.

I have the confidence now to not feel pressured or tempted into drinking or eating foods I don't want. Of course, there are times when I need to check in and see if my old habits are creeping back, but I'm aware now, and that gives me so much more control.

Char-grilled tuna steak with citrus salad

Ruby-red tuna steak really is spectacular. Make sure you don't overcook it and destroy the gorgeous colour and juicy texture!

SERVES 2 | **PREP** 15 minutes | **COOK** 5 minutes | **CAL PER SERVE** 306

1 ruby grapefruit, segmented
2 oranges, segmented
50 g baby rocket
2 teaspoons extra virgin olive oil

olive oil spray
250 g tuna steak
freshly ground black pepper

1. Combine the fruit segments, rocket and olive oil in a large bowl and gently toss to coat.

2. Preheat a char-grill or barbecue flat plate on high and lightly spray with olive oil. Season the tuna with pepper and cook for 2 minutes each side. Serve sliced with the salad.

TIP: You don't need the juice from the oranges or grapefruit for this salad, but don't waste it! Segment the fruit over a bowl and drink the juice that drips out as your aperitif while barbecuing the tuna.

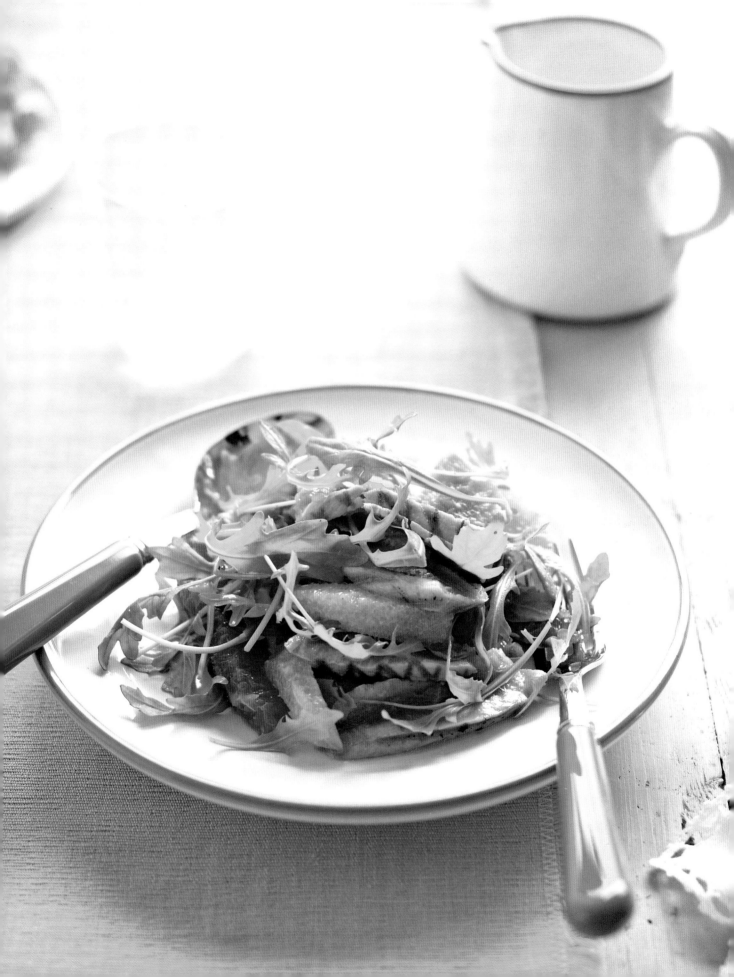

Salmon teriyaki with mushrooms and Asian greens

A classic Japanese-style dish that makes a fast and beautifully flavoursome weeknight dinner.

SERVES 2 | **PREP** 10 minutes | **COOK** 10 minutes | **CAL PER SERVE** 334

300 g salmon fillet, skin off
1½ tablespoons teriyaki sauce
1 teaspoon peanut oil
400 g mixed mushrooms
   (oyster, shiitake, swiss brown)

2 cloves garlic, crushed
1 bunch baby bok choy,
   leaves separated and washed

1. Place the salmon on a shallow plate and drizzle over the teriyaki sauce. Turn to coat.

2. Put a saucepan of water on to boil.

3. Heat the oil in a non-stick frying pan on high. Cook the mushrooms for 3–4 minutes, until they're tender and the moisture has evaporated. Stir through the garlic and cook for a further 15 seconds, then remove the garlicky mushrooms from the pan and keep warm.

4. In the same pan, cook the salmon for 1 minute each side (or until done to your liking). At the same time, steam the bok choy over the saucepan of boiling water until just wilted.

5. Serve the fish with a side of garlic mushrooms and steamed bok choy.

TIP: You can use whatever mushrooms you find while shopping. Leave oyster mushrooms whole, but cut the other mushrooms in half if they're large.

Snap out of it!

- If you eat more than your calorie quota you will NOT lose weight.

- Going to the gym three times a week doesn't mean you'll lose weight.

- Justification sentences like 'I deserve it' are childish,
  especially since you actually deserve better.

- Why are you eating like it's the Last Supper? Don't worry;
  we're not going to run out of food any time soon.

- So your parents/husband/friends are fat? It doesn't mean you have to be.

- There is no such thing as a fat gene.

- If you say you're going to clean up your act, the challenge won't be in the doing,
  it'll be in being your word. Once you are your word, it's actually easy.

- Quit looking for the quick fix! That butt of yours was a while in the making.

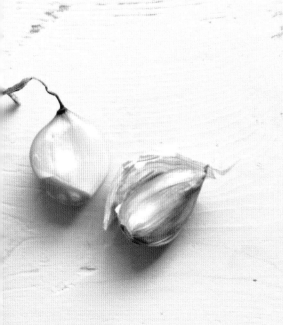

Thai fish burgers in lettuce cups

These burgers look amazing and taste just as good. You won't miss the bun.

SERVES 2 | **PREP** 25 minutes | **COOK** 20 minutes | **CAL PER SERVE** 268

400 g white fish fillet, skin off,
   deboned and cut into chunks
100 g green beans, finely chopped
1½ tablespoons Thai red curry paste
2 spring onions, finely chopped
2 tablespoons finely chopped
   coriander

½ teaspoon freshly ground
   black pepper
cooking oil spray
6 small iceberg lettuce leaves,
   trimmed into cups
½ Lebanese cucumber, shredded
2 tablespoons coriander sprigs
lime wedges, to serve

1. Using the pulse button on your food processor, process the fish very gently until just broken up. Transfer to a large bowl, add the beans, curry paste, spring onion, chopped coriander and pepper, and stir until well combined.

2. Lightly spray a non-stick frying pan with oil and heat on medium. Drop quarter-cups of the fish mixture into the pan to form burger patties, pressing each down lightly with the back of a spatula. Cook for 3–4 minutes each side until golden and cooked through.

3. Place the patties into the lettuce cups and top with the cucumber and coriander sprigs. Serve with lime wedges.

TIPS: Don't over-process the fish or the texture will be tough.

• You can make smaller or large burger patties depending on your preference. Wetting your hands with cold water will help prevent the fish mixture sticking to them.

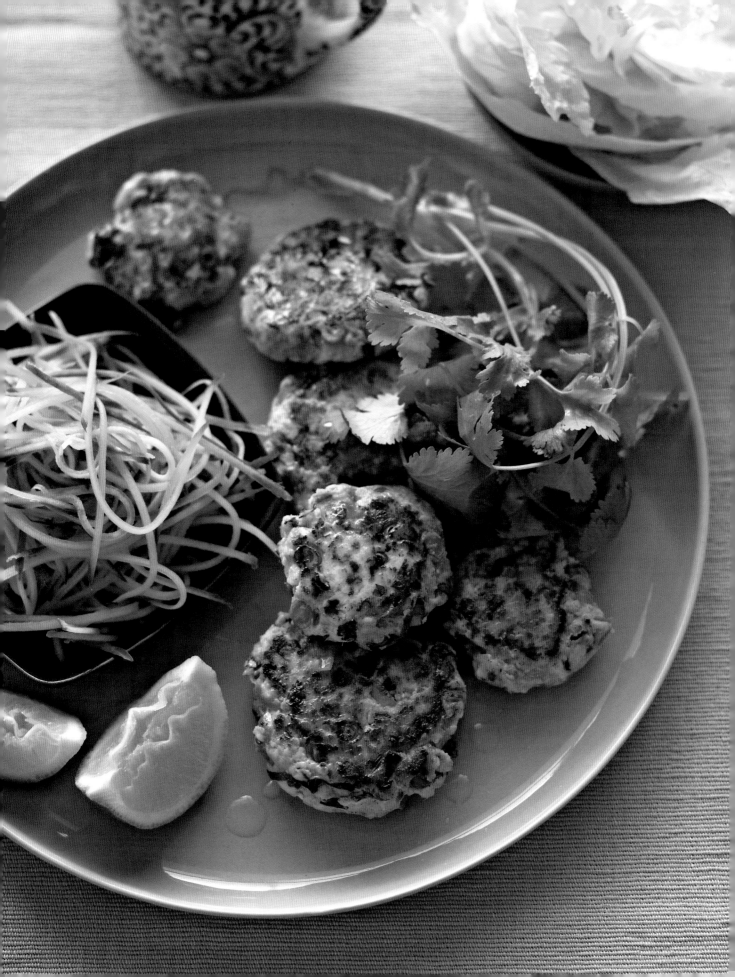

Char-grilled lamb and vegetable salad

Something a little different for the barbecue. The balsamic glaze isn't added until you assemble the salad, making for easy clean-up of your char-grill plate.

SERVES 2 | **PREP** 10 minutes | **COOK** 10 minutes | **CAL PER SERVE** 331

240 g lamb backstrap, trimmed
2 teaspoons olive oil
freshly ground black pepper
100 g baby rocket

2 red capsicums, trimmed
  and cut into wedges
1 large red onion, cut into wedges
1 tablespoon balsamic glaze

1. Heat a char-grill pan or barbecue on high.

2. Brush the lamb with a little of the olive oil, season with pepper and set aside. Wash the rocket if necessary and place in a large bowl.

3. In a separate bowl, toss the capsicum and onion with the remaining olive oil, then tip onto the hot pan or barbecue. Cook, stirring occasionally, for 10 minutes or until tender. Transfer them to a bowl, drizzle with the balsamic glaze, toss to coat, and place in the bowl with the rocket.

4. Towards the end of the vegetables' cooking time, add the lamb to the char-grill and cook for 2–3 minutes a side until well browned but still pink inside. Remove and stand for 5 minutes before slicing and adding to the salad. Toss gently to combine.

TIP: Balsamic glaze, or 'reduction', is available at your local supermarket. Not to be confused with plain balsamic vinegar, glaze is a thicker, stickier version that makes a great marinade.

Steak with garlic and anchovy dressing and mixed veggies

Really good organic and free-range steak is worth paying a bit more for. You'll definitely taste the difference.

SERVES 2 | PREP 15 minutes | COOK 5 minutes | CAL PER SERVE 323

300 g rump steak, trimmed of fat
freshly ground black pepper
olive oil spray
1 bunch broccolini
3 patty-pan squash, halved
100 g snowpeas, trimmed
1 zucchini, sliced on the diagonal

Garlic and anchovy dressing
1 tablespoon lemon juice
2 teaspoons extra virgin olive oil
3 anchovies in brine, drained
    and finely chopped
2 cloves garlic, crushed

1. Put a saucepan of water on to boil.

2. To make the dressing, combine all the ingredients in a small bowl.

3. Season the steak with pepper. Lightly spray a frying pan or char-grill with olive oil and heat on high, then cook the steak for 1 minute each side for rare (or until done to your liking).

4. Meanwhile, steam the broccolini and squash over the saucepan of boiling water for 2 minutes; add the snowpeas and zucchini and steam for another minute. Serve the steak and vegetables drizzled with the garlic and anchovy dressing.

Pork chop with cauliflower mash

I never used to eat pork, because I'm strict about *only* eating free-range meat and there just wasn't any. But now pork producers have stepped up to the plate. Otway Pork is one brand that provides free-range and humanely reared meat – you'll find the flavour an absolute revelation.

SERVES 2 | **PREP** 10 minutes | **COOK** 10 minutes | **CAL PER SERVE** 314

600 g cauliflower, broken into florets
olive oil spray
2 pork chops, trimmed of fat

½ cup low-cal ricotta
freshly ground black pepper
freshly grated nutmeg

1. Place the cauliflower in a microwave-safe bowl and microwave, covered, on high for 10 minutes or until tender.

2. Meanwhile, lightly spray a frying pan with olive oil and heat on medium–high. Turn the heat down to medium, add the pork chops and cook for 5 minutes on each side, until browned and just cooked through.

3. Put the cooked cauliflower in a food processor or blender with the ricotta, then puree until smooth and season with pepper and freshly grated nutmeg.

4. Serve the pork with the cauliflower mash.

TIP: The trick with pork is to *just* cook it – in order to be moist and juicy it should be ever so slightly pink inside.

Slow-cooked leg of lamb with Greek salad

This leg of lamb requires long, slow cooking but the prep is quick and easy – it's perfect for a weekend lunch with friends and family, as apart from basting the meat occasionally, you're free to relax and chat. And the leftovers are particularly good!

SERVES 6 | PREP 30 minutes | MARINATE 4 hours | COOK 3 hours
STAND 20 minutes | CAL PER SERVE 359

2 tablespoons lemon juice
1 tablespoon olive oil
3 cloves garlic, crushed
¼ cup chopped oregano leaves
1 kg leg of lamb, trimmed of fat

Greek salad
½ large cos lettuce, shredded
500 g ripe tomatoes, sliced

1 red capsicum, sliced
1 Lebanese cucumber, sliced
1 red onion, thinly sliced
75 g low-cal feta, crumbled
⅓ cup kalamata olives
1 teaspoon dried oregano
2 tablespoons cider vinegar
1½ tablespoons extra virgin olive oil
freshly ground black pepper

1. Combine the lemon juice, olive oil, garlic and oregano in a shallow dish, then add the lamb and turn to coat, rubbing the marinade into the meat. Refrigerate for 4 hours or overnight, turning the meat occasionally. Remove from the refrigerator 30 minutes before roasting.

2. Preheat your oven to 160°C. Place the lamb, the marinade and 2 tablespoons of water in a roasting dish just big enough to fit the meat snugly. Roast for 3 hours, basting regularly, then remove the dish from the oven and stand, loosely covered with foil, for 20 minutes.

3. Meanwhile, make the Greek salad. Arrange the lettuce, tomato, capsicum, cucumber and onion on a large platter and sprinkle with the feta, olives and oregano. Drizzle with vinegar and olive oil and season with pepper.

4. Carve the lamb and serve it with the Greek salad.

Moroccan lamb shanks with pumpkin and mint

Lemon, mint and broad beans add a different twist to slow-cooked lamb shanks.

SERVES 4 | PREP 30 minutes | COOK 1 hour 45 minutes | CAL PER SERVE 344

olive oil spray
4 frenched lamb shanks,
   trimmed of fat
1 teaspoon olive oil
1 brown onion, diced
2 cloves garlic, crushed
1 tablespoon finely grated ginger

1 tablespoon Moroccan seasoning
1¼ cups good-quality chicken stock
250 g frozen broad beans
750 g pumpkin, peeled, seeded
   and cut into large cubes
1 tablespoon lemon juice
¼ cup shredded mint leaves

1. Lightly spray a large casserole dish with olive oil and heat on your stovetop on medium–high. Cook the lamb shanks for about 8 minutes, turning occasionally, or until well browned all over. Remove from the dish and discard any juices.

2. Heat the olive oil in the dish on medium and cook the onion, stirring, for 5 minutes or until softened. Stir in the garlic and ginger and cook for 30 seconds or until fragrant, then stir in the seasoning. Return the lamb to the dish with the stock and bring to the boil. Reduce the heat and simmer, covered, for 1 hour 10 minutes.

3. Meanwhile, cook the broad beans in a small saucepan of boiling water for 2 minutes. Drain and rinse under cold water, then drain again. Discard the beans' outer skins.

4. Add the pumpkin to the lamb and cook, covered, for about 20 minutes or until the lamb is tender and the pumpkin is just tender. Stir in the broad beans, lemon juice and mint, and serve.

TIPS: The trick with the pumpkin is to remove the pan from the heat before it gets mushy. It will continue to cook in the sauce, even off the heat, and the 5 minutes you spend organising things for the table are usually enough to finish it off.

• See p. 50 for a recipe for homemade chicken stock. Really good stock will make all the difference in this dish!

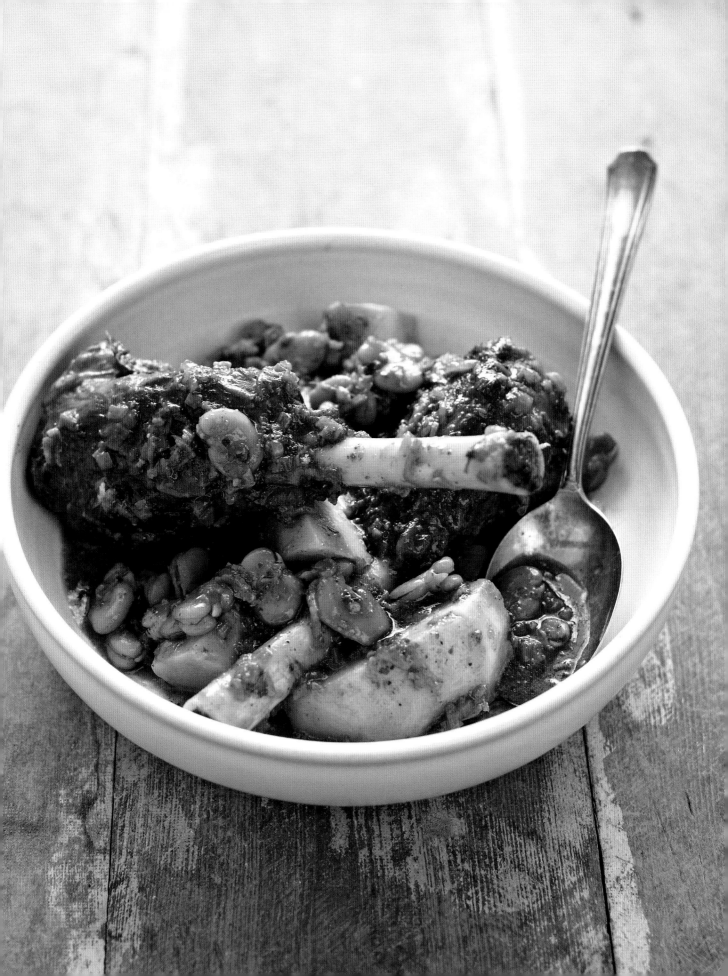

Pot-au-feu

I love a hearty, wholesome dish in cold weather. This is a great recipe for cheap cuts of beef such as blade or topside, which become very tender after slow-cooking.

SERVES 6 | PREP 15 minutes | COOK 2 hours 30 minutes | CAL PER SERVE 302

1 kg topside whole roast
1 brown onion, peeled
4 cloves
3 cloves garlic, peeled
1 stalk celery
8 parsley stems
1 bay leaf
4 sprigs fresh thyme
freshly ground black pepper

300 g carrots, peeled
    and cut into large chunks
300 g turnips, peeled and quartered
150 g parsnips, peeled
    and cut into large chunks
300 g sweet potato, peeled
    and cut into large chunks
6 pickling onions, peeled,
    leaving root intact
½ cup mustard, to serve

1. Combine the beef, onion, cloves, garlic, celery, parsley, bay leaf and thyme in a large heavy-based saucepan, and cover with 6 cups of water. Season with pepper and bring to the boil, then reduce the heat and simmer for 2 hours until the meat is tender.

2. Remove the beef from the pan. Using a fine sieve, strain the cooking liquid into a large bowl and discard the flavourings.

3. Return the strained broth to the pan with the beef, carrot, turnip, parsnip, sweet potato and pickling onions. Bring to the boil, reduce the heat and simmer for 30 minutes until the vegetables are tender.

4. Slice the beef very thinly and serve in shallow bowls with the vegetables and broth. Offer mustard on the side.

TIP: If your meat isn't in one compact piece, just tie it up like a roast with kitchen string.

Eggplant parmigiana

A healthy but delicious take on a classic dish. Terrific to cook ahead for the freezer, as well.

SERVES 5 | **PREP** 20 minutes | **COOK** 40 minutes | **CAL PER SERVE** 285

1 kg eggplant, trimmed
and thickly sliced
1 cup finely grated parmesan
1 cup grated mozzarella

2 cups tomato passata
½ cup coarsely chopped fresh oregano
2 cups fresh wholemeal breadcrumbs
80 g mixed salad leaves, to serve

1. Preheat your oven to 200°C.

2. Bring a large saucepan of water to the boil and steam the eggplant over it for 10 minutes until very soft. Drain on paper towel.

3. Combine the parmesan and mozzarella in a bowl.

4. Spread the base of a 5-cup capacity ovenproof dish with ½ cup of the passata. Layer with a third of the eggplant, a quarter of the cheese and 2 tablespoons of oregano, then repeat the layers twice. Finish with ½ cup of passata, the remaining cheese and the breadcrumbs, and bake for 30 minutes or until golden.

5. Serve with the mixed salad leaves.

TIP: If you're feeding four people you can divide this into four serves (356 cal per serve), or make the five serves and just keep the extra one to eat the next day for lunch – the flavours will have developed even further by then. To keep the topping crisp, pop your serving under the grill for a few minutes after you reheat it.

Baked spinach and pumpkin couscous

The couscous stays beautifully moist in this dish, as it steams under the layer of tomato passata.

SERVES 2 | **PREP** 15 minutes | **COOK** 40 minutes | **CAL PER SERVE** 311

olive oil spray
200 g pumpkin, peeled,
   seeded and sliced
½ cup couscous
40 g spinach, trimmed and shredded

⅔ cup tomato passata
1 clove garlic, crushed
freshly ground black pepper
⅓ cup finely grated parmesan

1. Preheat your oven to 200°C.

2. Lightly spray a char-grill with olive oil and heat on medium–high. Add the pumpkin and grill for 5 minutes on each side or until lightly charred and starting to soften. Dice into 2 cm cubes.

3. Meanwhile, place the couscous in a medium bowl and pour over half a cup of boiling water. Fluff the couscous up with a fork until most of the water has been absorbed, then cover and stand for 2 minutes. Fluff up with a fork again and stand, covered, for another 2 minutes. Stir through the spinach and pumpkin, then spoon the mixture into a 3-cup ovenproof dish and gently press down.

4. Combine the tomato passata and garlic in a bowl, and season with pepper. Cover the couscous with the tomato mixture and sprinkle with parmesan.

5. Bake for 30 minutes or until the cheese is melted and lightly browned.

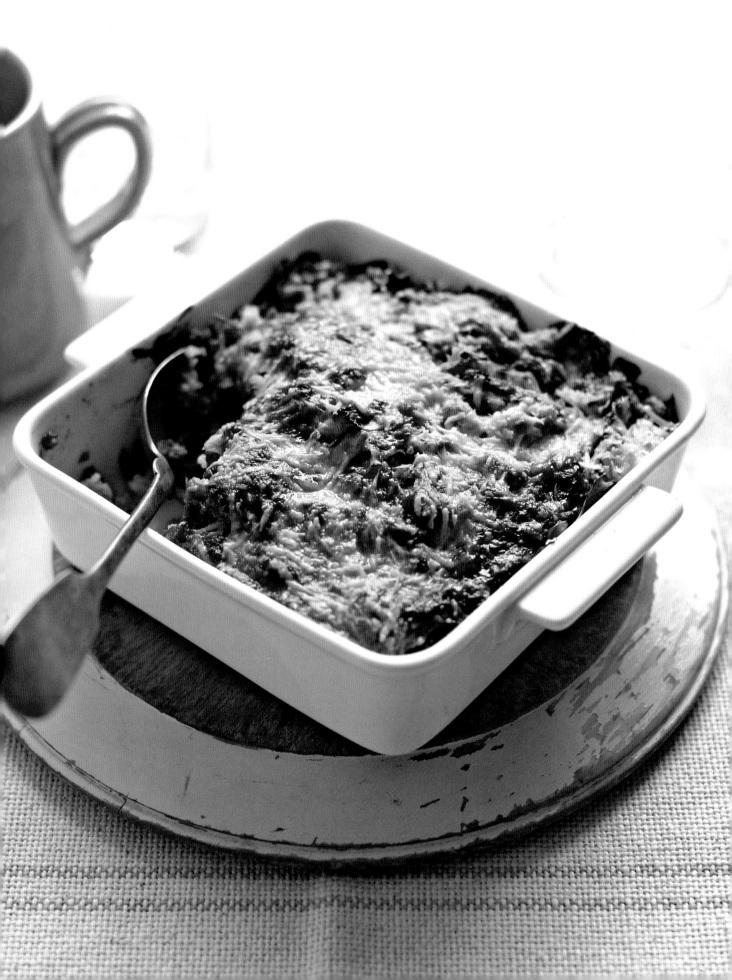

Mixed vegetable and cheese bake

With creamy ricotta, parmesan and melt-in-your-mouth
vegetables, what's not to like?

SERVES 4 | **PREP** 30 minutes | **COOK** 45 minutes | **CAL PER SERVE** 309

500 g celeriac, peeled
  and cut into 3 cm cubes
olive oil spray
500 g sweet potato, peeled
  and thinly sliced
1 teaspoon olive oil

1 leek, halved lengthwise
  and cut into 6 cm pieces
4 silverbeet leaves (green part only)
1½ cups low-cal ricotta
1 egg
½ cup finely grated parmesan
freshly ground black pepper

1. Preheat your oven to 200°C.

2. Place the celeriac in a microwave-safe
   bowl and microwave, covered, on high
   for 5 minutes until soft. Coarsely mash
   with a potato masher.

3. Meanwhile, lightly spray a large non-stick
   frying pan with olive oil and cook the sweet
   potato in batches for 3 minutes each side
   until softened. Remove and set aside.
   Heat the olive oil in the same frying pan and
   cook the leek for 3 minutes until softened.

4. Bring a medium saucepan of water to the
   boil, drop in the silverbeet leaves and cook
   for 30 seconds or until wilted. Drain and
   cool in ice-water, then drain well on
   paper towel and shred thinly.

5. In a medium bowl, combine the ricotta,
   the egg and all but 1 tablespoon of the
   parmesan; season with pepper.

6. Spread a third of the ricotta mixture over
   the base of a deep 5-cup ovenproof dish.
   Cover with half the leek, all the sweet
   potato and another third of the ricotta.
   Top with the silverbeet, celeriac and the
   remaining leek and ricotta. Sprinkle over
   the reserved parmesan and bake for
   30 minutes until golden and set.

TIP: You can also make this in four
1¼ cup-capacity deep ramekins – great
for the freezer or to put in a lunch box!

Pumpkin, onion and cinnamon pot pies

Feta, pumpkin and pine nuts are a match made in heaven. These little pies make a beautiful autumn dinner and can be on the table in 40 minutes flat. Great for lunch, too.

SERVES 2 | **PREP** 15 minutes | **COOK** 25 minutes | **CAL PER SERVE** 341

900 g pumpkin, peeled, seeded
  and cut into 1 cm slices
1 teaspoon olive oil
1 large brown onion, thinly sliced
pinch of ground cinnamon

freshly ground black pepper
40 g low-cal feta, crumbled
2 tablespoons pine nuts
1 tablespoon finely shredded mint

1. Preheat your oven to 220°C.

2. Place the pumpkin in a microwave-safe bowl, cover, and microwave on high for 8 minutes or until tender. Coarsely mash with a potato masher.

3. Meanwhile, heat the olive oil in a frying pan on medium–high and cook the onion, stirring, for 10 minutes until well browned and tender. Reduce the heat to low and cook, covered, for a further 5 minutes, then remove from the heat. Stir in the cinnamon and season with pepper.

4. Spread the base of two shallow 1¼ cup-capacity ramekins with half of the pumpkin. Top with the onion and the remaining pumpkin, then sprinkle over the feta and pine nuts. Bake for 10 minutes and serve sprinkled with mint.

Roasted Mediterranean vegetables

This rustic vegetable bake looks gorgeous and tastes just as good. You'll love the steamed eggplant, which is absolutely luscious without tons of oil clogging it up.

SERVES 2 | **PREP** 30 minutes | **COOK** 1 hour 25 minutes | **CAL PER SERVE** 354

400 g eggplant, sliced into rounds
2 cups fresh wholemeal breadcrumbs
⅓ cup finely chopped parsley
1 tablespoon finely chopped
   fresh thyme
2 teaspoons olive oil
1 clove garlic, crushed

300 g roma tomatoes,
   sliced into rounds
2 zucchini, thinly sliced into rounds
1 brown onion, halved and thinly
   sliced into rounds
1 large red capsicum, cut into chunks
¼ cup pitted kalamata olives, sliced

1. Preheat your oven to 200°C.

2. Bring a saucepan of water to the boil and steam the eggplant over it for 10 minutes or until soft. Drain on paper towel.

3. Sprinkle half the breadcrumbs into a 4½ cup-capacity ovenproof dish. Bake for 5 minutes until the crumbs are lightly toasted.

4. Combine the remaining breadcrumbs with the herbs, olive oil and garlic in a medium bowl.

5. In your ovenproof dish, arrange the steamed eggplant and rounds of tomato, zucchini, onion and capsicum on their edges in tight alternating rows on top of the toasted breadcrumbs (say, one row of zucchini rounds standing on their edges, pressed flat against the side of the dish, then one row of eggplant on end, flat against the zucchini, and so on). Push olives randomly down between the vegetables, sprinkle the herbed breadcrumb mixture over the top, and cover the bake with foil.

6. Cook in the oven for 45 minutes, then uncover and bake for another 25 minutes or until the vegetables are tender and the breadcrumbs are golden and crisp.

TIPS: To make the rows neat, try to slice the vegetables so that they're all roughly the same size.

• This is a terrific side dish for grilled rump steak (to serve 4, with 125 g trimmed steak per person, it's 338 cal per serve) or for grilled fish (330 cal per serve for a 150 g white fish fillet per person).

Jo from Kaimkillenbun, 28

Starting weight: 109 kg

At the time of writing: 82 kg

All I ate was crap! Junk food. All the time! Lots of take-out; as soon as I finished work I would load up and hit the couch. No fruit, no vegetables unless you count potato chips, no water. I only ever drank soft drink or cordial. I would regularly eat an entire pizza with garlic bread and a bottle of soft drink for dinner. That one meal would be close to two days' eating for me now.

I had thyroid cancer in 2007, and I was at my heaviest weight of 115 kg. Once my thyroid was removed, I was told I had to lose weight, which I did. I got down to where I am now: 82 kg. Then my dad passed away and I just gave up. I turned to food. It was emotional, comfort eating. I didn't cook, I didn't care. I tried a couple of diets, but I never stuck to them.

With Michelle's plan, I simply did everything she told me to do. I went completely cold turkey and with her support I just hung in there. The first week I had the shakes, headaches and I threw up every time I exercised – I had the full withdrawal symptoms. My body was completely detoxing itself, it was crazy.

I now cook all my meals. I only drink water; I eat fresh fruit and vegetables. All my meals are between 300 and 350 calories and I just have a piece of fruit if I want a snack. It's so simple really, when you think about it. And I'm literally bursting with energy! I sleep better: I just feel amazing! I also have more money – it was expensive eating so much and always buying take-out.

I absolutely have my life back. I have Jo back and I'm the happiest I've ever been. Dad would be so proud.

Moroccan roasted chicken with spiced carrot salad

I love a roast, and a roast with lots of spices is even better. It's the ultimate soul food.

SERVES 6 | **PREP** 15 minutes | **COOK** 1 hour | **CAL PER SERVE** 354

1.6 kg whole chicken, skin removed
olive oil spray
freshly ground black pepper
1 lemon, halved
1 tablespoon Moroccan seasoning
½ cup coarsely chopped parsley

Spiced carrot salad
1.2 kg carrots, peeled and
  cut into 1.5 cm slices
1½ tablespoons extra virgin olive oil
1 teaspoon cumin seeds
½ teaspoon ground coriander
½ teaspoon paprika
1 teaspoon harissa
¼ cup lemon juice
⅓ cup coarsely chopped mint

1. Preheat your oven to 200°C.

2. Pat the chicken dry with paper towel, then lightly spray it with olive oil and season with pepper. Squeeze a half lemon over it and rub in the seasoning. Squeeze the juice of the remaining lemon half into the chicken cavity, then place both lemon halves inside with the parsley. Season the cavity with pepper. Truss the chicken with kitchen string and place on a wire rack on a roasting tray. Roast for 1 hour, basting regularly, until the chicken juices run clear when you pierce the thickest part with a skewer. Stand, loosely covered, for 5 minutes before carving.

3. Meanwhile, to make the salad, put the carrots into a large saucepan and barely cover them with water. Bring to the boil, then reduce the heat and simmer for 8–10 minutes until they're tender but still have a crunch. Drain well and place in a large bowl.

4. Heat the olive oil in a small frying pan on medium. Add the spices and harissa and cook, stirring, until fragrant. Pour the mixture over the carrots, along with the lemon juice, and gently toss to coat. When the carrots have cooled slightly, toss through the mint.

5. Serve the chicken with the spiced carrots.

TIPS: If you leave the skin on the chicken, this has 431 cal per serve!

• Due to the seasoning, the chicken will take on quite a dark brown colour – don't panic, just test for doneness by piercing with a skewer as normal.

• The salad improves if left to stand at room temperature for 1–2 hours.

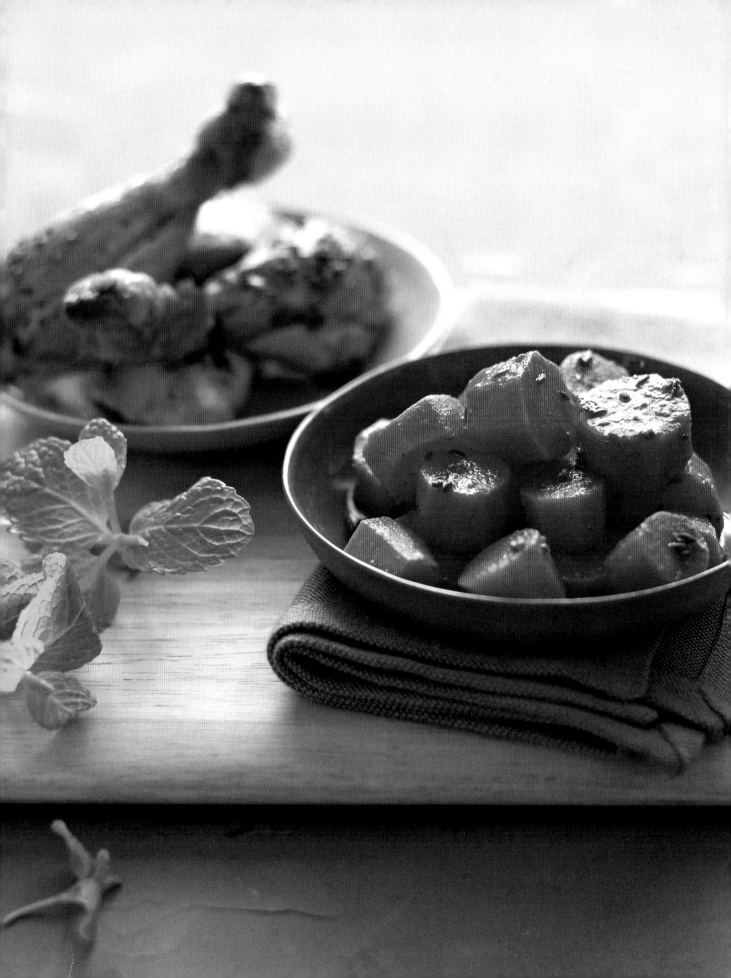

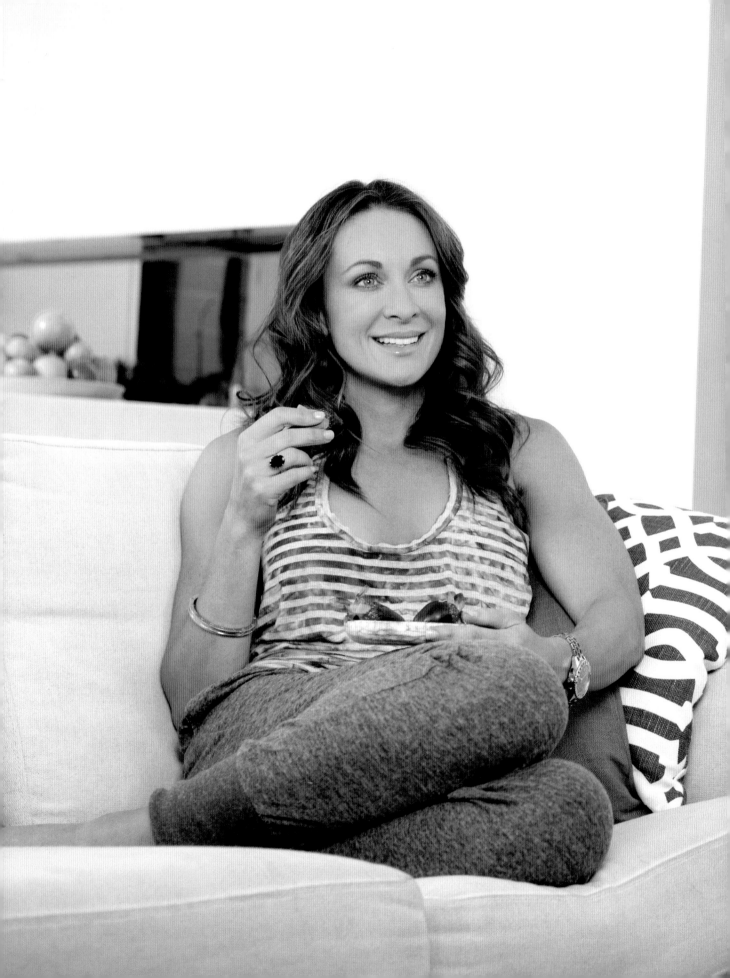

dessert

Chocolate strawberries

These are so simple, but absolutely delicious. They make a showstopping dessert for a dinner party, or a romantic addition to a picnic for two.

SERVES 4 | **PREP** 10 minutes | **COOK** 5 minutes | **CHILL** 30 minutes | **CAL PER SERVE** 133

80 g dark chocolate
500 g strawberries

1. Bring a saucepan of water to the boil, then reduce the heat to a simmer. Place a heatproof bowl over the saucepan (make sure the water doesn't touch the bowl), add the chocolate, and allow to melt.

2. Holding the strawberries by the calyx (the green leaves around the top), dip them in chocolate and place them on a tray lined with baking paper. Chill in the refrigerator until set.

TIP: Don't wash the strawberries, simply brush them lightly with paper towel if you think they need it.

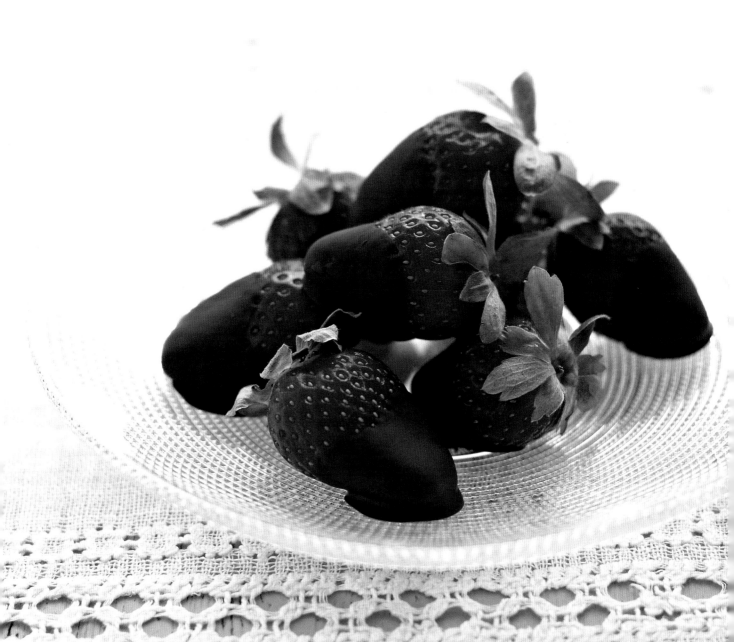

Date and ricotta tarts

Dates and ricotta are a winning combination wherever you put them. The filo pastry has a lovely rustic look and a wonderful crunch – and is low in calories!

SERVES 4 | **PREP** 10 minutes | **COOK** 20 minutes | **CAL PER SERVE** 152

3 sheets filo pastry
olive oil spray
1 teaspoon ground cinnamon
½ cup low-cal ricotta

100 g dates, seeded and thinly sliced
2 Valencia oranges
1 tablespoon small mint leaves

1. Preheat your oven to 180°C, and line a baking tray with baking paper.

2. Lightly spray each sheet of filo pastry with olive oil and sprinkle over a little cinnamon. Arrange two sheets on top of each other and cut into quarters to make four rectangles of pastry for the bases.

3. Cut the remaining pastry sheet into quarters, then fold each rectangle in half and in half again. Place one of these in the centre of each two-layer tart base, to strengthen it.

4. Spread the ricotta over the centre of the pastry bases and top with the dates, then spray the edges of the pastry with olive oil and roughly fold over to form a thicker frame around the filling. Sprinkle the tarts with the remaining cinnamon and place on your prepared tray. Bake for 20 minutes until the pastry is golden and crisp.

5. Meanwhile, peel the oranges, cutting away the rind and pith. Slice the peeled oranges thinly.

6. Place each filo tart on a plate, arrange a few orange slices on the side and sprinkle with mint. Serve immediately.

TIP: Filo pastry dries out very rapidly and becomes too brittle to work with, so you need to work quickly once you have opened the packet. Keep the remaining sheets covered with a damp cloth and then store them in the refrigerator wrapped in plastic film.

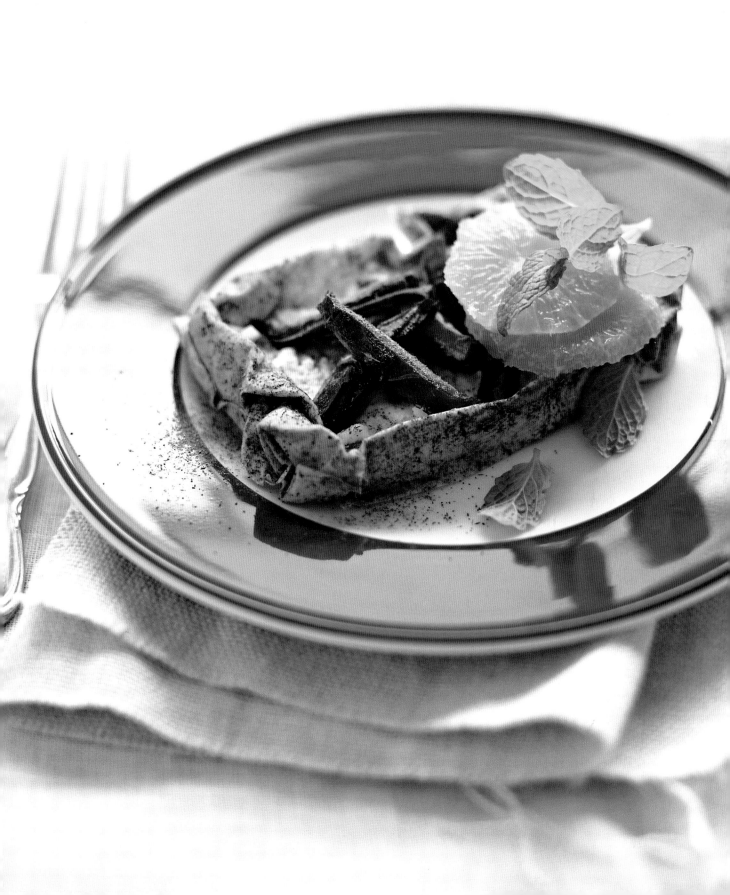

Pear and ginger crumble

The ginger in this crumble really gives it a zing and makes
it the perfect dessert for cold winter nights.

SERVES 4 | PREP 10 minutes | COOK 25 minutes | CAL PER SERVE 152

cooking oil spray
500 g ripe pears, peeled,
    cored and cut into small chunks
20 g uncrystallised candied ginger,
    finely chopped

⅔ cup low-sugar untoasted muesli
⅔ cup plain low-cal yoghurt

1. Preheat your oven to 200°C and lightly spray
   four half-cup capacity ramekins with oil.

2. Place the pear and ginger in a large bowl
   and toss, then divide between the ramekins
   and top with the muesli. Bake for
   25 minutes until golden.

3. Serve warm with a dollop of yoghurt.

Fruit salad

Fruit salad is such a classic, and it's terrific for breakfast as well as dessert. This is great to make in advance – you could even make enough for a week and store it in the fridge. Just make sure you take it out a little before you eat it, as the flavours will be stronger at room temperature.

SERVES 4 | PREP 15 minutes | CAL PER SERVE 148

1 passionfruit
500 g rockmelon, peeled, seeded
    and cut into chunks
500 g honeydew melon, peeled,
    seeded and cut into chunks

1 small mango, peeled,
    stoned and cubed
150 g seedless green grapes,
    halved if large

1. Cut the passionfruit in half and scoop out the pulp, then stir through the remaining ingredients. Serve in small bowls.

TIP: You need about ¼ cup of passionfruit pulp for this recipe, so if the passionfruit is small you may want to use two.

Blueberry millefeuilles

Blueberries are chock-full of antioxidants and vitamins – though when you eat these decadent millefeuilles, I guarantee you won't be thinking anything but how good they taste.

SERVES 4 | **PREP** 20 minutes | **COOK** 5 minutes | **CAL PER SERVE** 150

cooking oil spray
4 sheets filo pastry
400 g blueberries

⅔ cup vanilla frûche
1 teaspoon icing sugar (optional)

1. Preheat the oven to 200°C. Lightly spray two baking trays with oil.

2. Layer the filo sheets on top of one another, spraying each layer with oil, and press down. Cut the stack in half lengthwise, then cut each half into eight rectangles – you'll have four spare in case you break any. Place them on the prepared tray and bake for 2–3 minutes until golden. Allow to cool.

3. Reserve ½ cup of blueberries.

4. Place four pastry rectangles onto dessert plates. Spread 1 tablespoon of frûche onto each rectangle, top with berries and repeat the filo, frûche and berries to form a second layer. Finish with another piece of filo and sprinkle with icing sugar, if using.

5. Scatter the reserved berries around the millefeuille and serve immediately.

TIPS: You need to assemble the millefeuilles just before serving or the filo pastry will go soggy.

• To prevent the millefeuille skidding around the plate, place a dab of frûche under the first rectangle of filo.

• This is also lovely made with raspberries, or with mixed raspberries and blueberries.

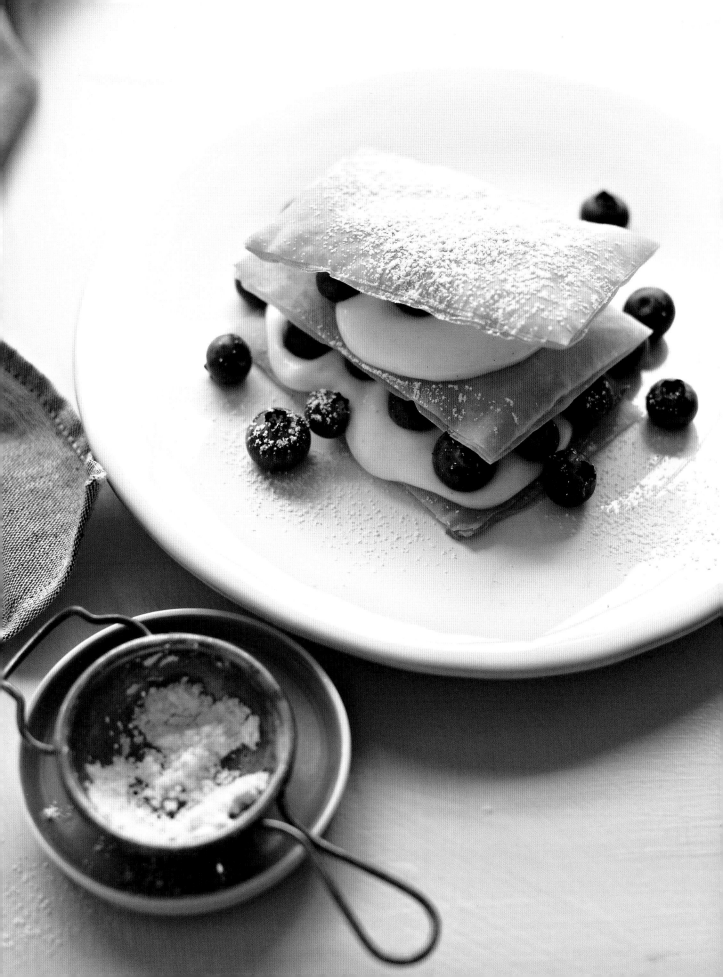

Sugar-grilled tropical salad

There's nothing like grilling fruit to bring out the sweetness and make an everyday food into something really special. Kids go nuts for this tropical platter.

SERVES 4 | **PREP** 10 minutes | **COOK** 5 minutes | **CAL PER SERVE** 133

500 g pineapple, peeled
  and thickly sliced
2 medium mangoes
2 teaspoons brown sugar

2 passionfruit, halved
1 star fruit, sliced
1 lime, quartered

1. Preheat a char-grill on medium–high, then grill the pineapple for 1–2 minutes each side until charred.

2. Meanwhile, halve the mangoes, cutting each along both sides of the stone. Discard the stones and, using a small sharp knife, cut the flesh inside in a crisscross pattern, taking care not to pierce the skin. Sprinkle each mango half with a little brown sugar and grill flesh-side down for 1 minute until lightly charred.

3. Divide the warm char-grilled pineapple and mango between four dessert plates, along with the remaining fruit. Squeeze the lime over the mango to serve.

Apple, blueberry and cinnamon crepes

Frozen pre-prepared crepes make this dessert super-easy and help you keep the portion size under control – we like the Creative Gourmet brand. But if you're feeling inspired, go ahead and make your own crepes from scratch! Just watch the calorie count in the recipe you choose: the Creative Gourmet crepes have 102 cal each.

SERVES 4 | PREP 10 minutes | COOK 10 minutes | CAL PER SERVE 149

cooking oil spray
2 large pink lady apples, peeled, cored and cut into 1 cm thick wedges

100 g blueberries
pinch of cinnamon, plus extra to serve
4 frozen French-style crepes

1. Lightly spray a non-stick frying pan with oil and heat on medium–high. Cook the apples for 8 minutes, covered, until golden and tender, turning halfway through. Remove from the heat, add the blueberries and sprinkle with cinnamon.

2. Warm the crepes according to the packet directions and place them on four warmed dessert plates. Divide the apple mixture between them, placing the fruit on one side and folding each crepe over to enclose. Serve immediately with a pinch of cinnamon on top.

TIP: Make sure you use a frying pan that's big enough to fit all the apples in one layer, so they cook evenly.

Strawberries with balsamic and orange glaze

This is another fantastic dessert for entertaining. You can plate up the berries well beforehand, then drizzle them with dressing just before serving. Too easy!

SERVES 4 | **PREP** 10 minutes | **CAL PER SERVE** 127

500 g small strawberries
1 tablespoon balsamic glaze
   (see note on p. 110)
1 tablespoon orange juice

zest of half an orange,
   cut into matchsticks
¼ cup small basil leaves
1 cup vanilla frûche

1. Hull the strawberries and cut a third of them in half, then place them on a platter. Combine the balsamic glaze and orange juice and drizzle over the berries. Sprinkle with the zest and basil leaves.

2. Serve the strawberries with a bowl of vanilla frûche for your guests to help themselves.

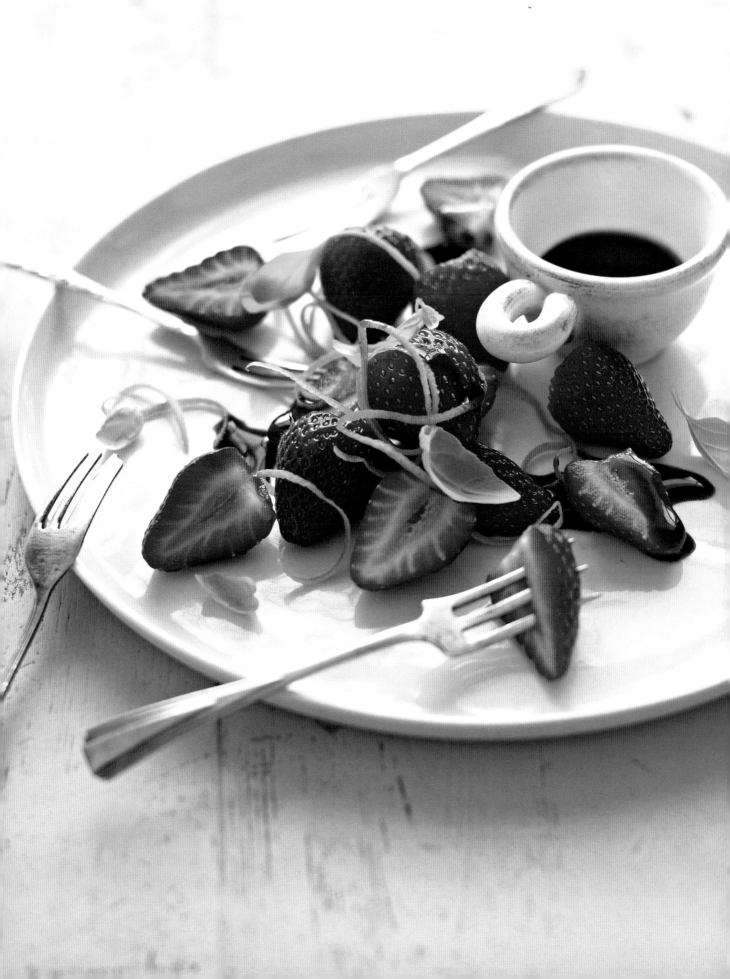

Using the menu plans

Each dish in this book has around 250 to 350 calories per serve, so adding a snack or two to these menus (from the list on page 43) will give you a daily quota of around 1200 calories – perfect for the girls. Guys need to add a serve of rice or pasta or a slice of wholegrain bread, to make it up to between 1300 and 1600 calories.

If you don't need to lose weight, you can add an extra snack plus half a cup of cooked rice or pasta to one meal, to reach around 1500 calories for girls and 1800 calories for guys. But if you start putting on kilos, cut back!

Food essentials

Here's a guide to the basics you'll need to have in the pantry, fridge and freezer to make cooking fuss-free each week.

All-Bran

anchovies in brine

bread: mixed-grain, Mountain Bread, rye and wholemeal

broad beans, frozen

brown rice, medium-grain

bulgur (cracked wheat)

canned beans: cannellini beans and chickpeas

canned beetroot

canned tuna in springwater

couscous

dried fruit: currants and sultanas

eggs

flour: self-raising and wholemeal

garlic

ginger, fresh

harissa

herbs and spices: bay leaves, chilli, ground cinnamon, cloves, ground coriander, cumin seeds, ground cumin, curry powder, Moroccan seasoning, whole nutmeg, dried oregano, paprika and za'atar

lemons

lentils, brown

milk, low-cal

mustard: Dijon and wholegrain

nuts: pine nuts and walnuts

olive oil and olive oil spray, plus extra virgin olive oil for salad dressings

olives in brine

onions: brown and red

pasta, dried

peanut oil

peppercorns, whole black

rolled oats

sauces: fish sauce, hoisin sauce, oyster sauce, low-salt soy sauce, Tabasco and teriyaki sauce

shredded coconut

stock, chicken, low-salt

sugar: brown and icing

tomato passata

vegetable oil spray

vinegar: cider, malt, red-wine, sherry, white balsamic and white-wine

yoghurt, plain, low-cal

Weet-Bix

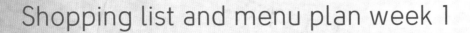

Shopping list and menu plan week 1

apple, green
asparagus
banana
basil
beans, green
beef, rump steak
black mustard seeds
bok choy, baby
breadstick
broccolini
capsicum, red
carrots
celery
cheddar, low-cal
chicken breast fillets
chicken, whole
chilli, long green
cranberry sauce
cucumbers, Lebanese
curry leaves, fresh
dates

dill
eggplant
feta, low-cal
figs, dried
filo pastry
grapefruit, ruby
grapes, seedless
honeydew melon
kangaroo fillet
lamb shanks, frenched
lettuce: whole iceberg
    and baby cos leaves
mint
mozzarella
oranges, valencia
oregano, fresh
parmesan
parsley, flat-leaf
passionfruit
pear
potatoes, kipfler

prunes, pitted
pumpkin
ricotta, low-cal
rocket
rockmelon
salad leaves, mixed
shallots, red
snowpeas
spinach, baby
spring onions
squash, patty-pan
tandoori seasoning
tofu, firm
tomatoes: large
    and roma
tuna steak
turkey, shaved
turkey, thinly sliced
    cooked
zucchini

The ●● symbols means you need to make extra for leftovers;
the ● symbol means you're using leftovers.

	breakfast	lunch	dinner	total cals
monday	Sweet couscous with orange juice and dried fruit, p. 4 353 cal	Cucumber, feta and za'atar roll, p. 21 277 cal	Pepper kangaroo stir-fry, p. 89 310 cal	940 + 260 cal for snacks
tuesday	All-Bran fruit salad, p. 6 350 cal	Turkey and cranberry sandwich, p. 19 323 cal	Char-grilled tuna steak with citrus salad, p. 104 306 cal	979 + 221 cal for snacks
wednesday	Morning Weet-Bix and passionfruit trifle, p. 3 342 cal	Tandoori chicken with carrot salad, p. 40 319 cal	Moroccan vegetable and couscous salad, p. 100 299 cal	960 + 240 cal for snacks
thursday	Turkey and egg toastie, p. 10 335 cal	Potato and egg salad with green beans and celery, p. 30 308 cal	●● Pumpkin, onion and cinnamon pot pies, p. 121 341 cal	984 + 216 cal for snacks
friday	Apple and pear porridge with cinnamon, p. 7 332 cal	● Pumpkin, onion and cinnamon pot pies, p. 121 341 cal	Steak with garlic and anchovy dressing and mixed veggies, p. 111 323 cal	996 + 204 cal for snacks
saturday	White beans with spinach on toast, p. 8 342 cal	Asparagus, rocket and ricotta frittata, p. 70 273 cal	Eggplant parmigiana, p. 117 285 cal + Date and ricotta tarts, p. 130 152 cal	1052 + 148 cal for snacks
sunday	Omelette stir-fry with tofu and bok choy, p. 11 357 cal	Greek lamb shanks with lentils, p. 59 355 cal	Moroccan roasted chicken with spiced carrot salad, p. 124 354 cal	1066 + 134 cal for snacks

Shopping list and menu plan week 2

apples: green and red

asparagus

banana

basil

beef, roast

beef, rump steak

blue cheese, sharp

bok choy, baby

breadstick

broccolini

buttermilk

celeriac

cheddar, low-cal

chicken breast fillets

chicken thigh fillets

chives

chocolate, dark

coriander, fresh

cottage cheese, low-cal

endive

figs, dried

flour: self-raising and
   wholemeal

gai lan

grapes, seedless

honeydew melon

lamb shanks, frenched

leeks

limes

mesclun salad mix

mint

miso, red

mushrooms, mixed

mussels

oranges

parmesan

passionfruit

pear

prunes, pitted

pumpkin

ricotta, low-cal

rockmelon

smoked salmon

spinach, baby

spring onions

star anise

strawberries

sweet corn, baby

sweet corn, cob

tarragon, fresh

tofu, firm

tomatoes: roma
   and mixed cherry

turkey, shaved

udon noodles

wine, dry white

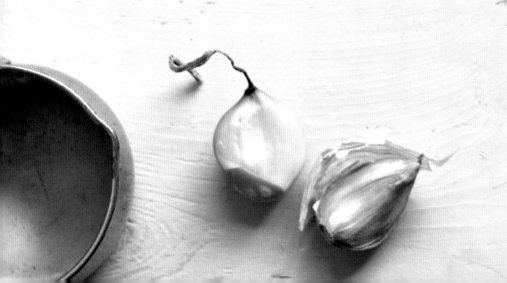

The ❤❤ symbols means you need to make extra for leftovers;
the ❤ symbol means you're using leftovers.

	breakfast	lunch	dinner	total cals
monday	Apple and pear porridge with cinnamon, p. 7 332 cal	Egg and tarragon sandwich, p. 16 320 cal	Beef and oyster sauce stir-fry, p. 92 343 cal	995 + 205 cal for snacks
tuesday	Morning Weet-Bix and passionfruit trifle, p. 3 342 cal	Celeriac coleslaw and rare roast beef sandwich, p. 22 303 cal	Leek and tarragon mussels, p. 85 355 cal	1000 + 200 cal for snacks
wednesday	Sweet couscous with orange juice and dried fruit, p. 4 353 cal	Chicken and udon noodle soup, p. 50 275 cal	Endive, walnut, blue cheese and apple salad, p. 76 310 cal	938 + 262 cal for snacks
thursday	All-Bran fruit salad, p. 6 350 cal	Smoked salmon and strawberry salad, p. 25 313 cal	❤❤ Baked spinach and pumpkin couscous, p. 118 311 cal	974 + 226 cal for snacks
friday	Turkey and egg toastie, p. 10 335 cal	❤ Baked spinach and pumpkin couscous, p. 118 311 cal	Miso chicken skewers with steamed Asian veggies, p. 88 289 cal	935 + 265 cal for snacks
saturday	Omelette stir-fry with tofu and bok choy, p. 11 357 cal	Tomato and basil pasta salad, p. 33 320 cal	❤❤ Moroccan lamb shanks with pumpkin and mint, p. 114 344 cal + Chocolate strawberries, p. 128 133 cal	1154 + 46 cal for snacks
sunday	Corn fritters, p. 12 357 cal	❤ Moroccan lamb shanks with pumpkin and mint, p. 114 344 cal	Warm roasted tomato salad, p. 77 227 cal	928 + 272 cal for snacks

Shopping list and menu plan week 3

apple, green
asparagus
balsamic glaze
banana
basil
bok choy, baby
broccolini
cabbage, red
capsicums: green
  and red
carrots
cheddar, low-cal
chicken breast fillets
chicken mince, lean
chives
coriander, fresh
cucumber, Lebanese
eggplant
fennel
feta, low-cal

figs, dried
ginger, uncrystallised
  candied
grapes, seedless
honeydew melon
lamb, backstrap
lamb, leg
lemongrass stalk
lettuce: cos and
  iceberg
limes
mint
muesli, low-sugar,
  untoasted
mushrooms, mixed
naan
oranges
oregano, fresh
parmesan
parsley, flat-leaf

passionfruit
pears
pita pockets,
  wholemeal
prawns, green
prunes, pitted
rocket, baby
rockmelon
salmon fillets
shallots, red
silverbeet
spinach, baby
spring onions
Thai basil
thyme, fresh
tofu, firm
tomatoes: large,
  cherry and roma
turkey, shaved
zucchini

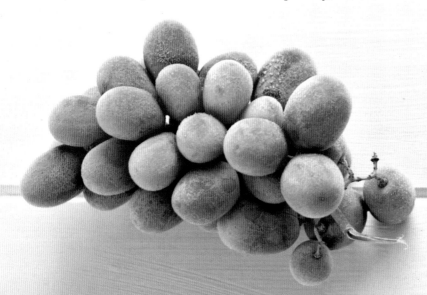

The ●● symbols means you need to make extra for leftovers;
the ● symbol means you're using leftovers.

	breakfast	lunch	dinner	total cals
monday	Apple and pear porridge with cinnamon, p. 7 332 cal	Lamb and tabouli pockets, p. 20 299 cal	Thai chilli prawn stir-fry, p. 84 246 cal	877 + 323 cal for snacks
tuesday	All-Bran fruit salad, p. 6 350 cal	Tuna, chickpea and coriander salad, p. 28 334 cal	Salmon teriyaki with mushrooms and Asian greens, p. 106 334 cal	1018 + 182 cal for snacks
wednesday	Sweet couscous with orange juice and dried fruit, p. 4 353 cal	White bean, tomato and basil salad, p. 37 300 cal	Thai chicken larb, p. 86 301 cal	954 + 246 cal for snacks
thursday	Morning Weet-Bix and passionfruit trifle, p. 3 342 cal	Chicken, beetroot and mint sandwich, p. 24 299 cal	●● Roasted Mediterranean vegetables, p. 122 354 cal	995 + 205 cal for snacks
friday	Turkey and egg toastie, p. 10 335 cal	● Roasted Mediterranean vegetables, p. 122 354 cal	Char-grilled lamb and vegetable salad, p. 110 331 cal	1020 + 180 cal for snacks
saturday	White beans with spinach on toast, p. 8 342 cal	Zucchini and curry soup, p. 49 280 cal	Slow-cooked leg of lamb with Greek salad, p. 113 359 cal + Pear and ginger crumble, p. 132 152 cal	1133 + 67 cal for snacks
sunday	Omelette stir-fry with tofu and bok choy, p. 11 357 cal	●● Lebanese lentil soup, p. 48 305 cal	'Rainbow' fried brown rice, p. 91 316 cal	978 + 222 cal for snacks

Shopping list and menu plan week 4

apple, green
asparagus
avocado
banana
beef, rump steak
beef, topside whole
  roast
blueberries
bok choy, baby
capsicums: green
  and red
carrots
cauliflower
celeriac
celery
cheddar, low-cal
chicken breast fillets
chicken, whole
chives
coriander, fresh
corncob

cucumbers: Lebanese
  and long
fennel
figs, dried
filo pastry
frûche, vanilla
gai lan
grapes, seedless
honeydew melon
leek
lemongrass stalk
lettuce, iceberg
mango
mint
onions, pickling
oranges
parmesan
parsley, flat-leaf
parsnips
passionfruit
pear

pork chops
prawns, king, cooked
prunes, pitted
pumpkin
rice vermicelli noodles
ricotta, low-cal
rockmelon
salmon fillet, skin off
silverbeet
spring onions
sweet potatoes
thyme, fresh
tofu, firm
tomatoes, large
turkey, shaved
turnips
Vietnamese dipping
  sauce
water chestnuts,
  canned
watercress

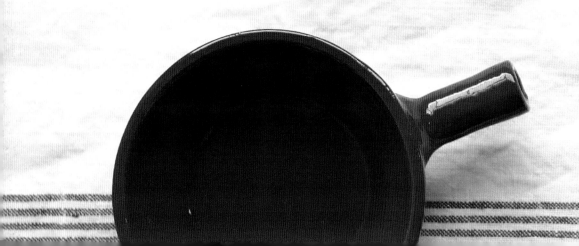

The ●● symbols means you need to make extra for leftovers;
the ● symbol means you're using leftovers.

	breakfast	lunch	dinner	total cals
monday	All-Bran fruit salad, p. 6 350 cal	● Lebanese lentil soup, p. 48 305 cal	●● Hoisin chicken, pumpkin and celery stir-fry, p. 94 331 cal	986 + 214 cal for snacks
tuesday	Turkey and egg toastie, p. 10 335 cal	Orange and watercress salad, p. 39 325 cal	Salmon stir-fry with gai lan and water chestnuts, p. 82 291 cal	951 + 249 cal for snacks
wednesday	Sweet couscous with orange juice and dried fruit, p. 4 353 cal	● Hoisin chicken, pumpkin and celery stir-fry, p. 94 331 cal	Prawn, mango and avocado salad, p. 74 321 cal	1005 + 195 cal for snacks
thursday	Apple and pear porridge with cinnamon, p. 7 332 cal	Watercress, fennel and parmesan salad, p. 36 271 cal	●● Mixed vegetable and cheese bake, p. 120 309 cal	912 + 288 cal for snacks
friday	Morning Weet-Bix and passionfruit trifle, p. 3 342 cal	● Mixed vegetable and cheese bake, p. 120 309 cal	Pork chop with cauliflower mash, p. 112 314 cal	965 + 235 cal for snacks
saturday	Corn fritters, p. 12 357 cal	Gazpacho, p. 46 252 cal	Pot-au-feu, p. 116 302 cal + Blueberry millefeuilles, p. 134 150 cal	1061 + 139 cal for snacks
sunday	Omelette stir-fry with tofu and bok choy, p. 11 357 cal	Vietnamese beef salad, p. 42 339 cal	Portuguese chicken with grilled capsicum salad, p. 96 326 cal	1022 + 178 cal for snacks

Index